MW00472749

"Burt Dragin has delivered the compulsive gambler's sourcebook, a detailed, troubling account of a family passion for the losing bet. *Six to Five Against* is funny and touching, full of compassion, brimming with detail that'll make any gambler wince with recognition, and steeped in foreboding. If you gamble more often that you want to (gamblers will understand this paradox), read this book. It won't make you stop gambling but you'll know you're not alone, and you'll be a lot more aware of what you're doing when you're doing it, which is one of the few tunnels out."

—Frederick Barthelme
Author of *Bob the Gambler*
and co-author of *Double Down*

SIX TO FIVE AGAINST

A Gambler's Odyssey

Burt Dragin

RDR Books
Berkeley, California

Six to Five Against

RDR Books
2415 Woolsey
Berkeley, CA 94705
Phone: (510) 595-0595
Fax: (510) 228-0300
E-mail: Read@rdrbooks.com
Website: www.rdrbooks.com

Copyright 2005 by Burt Dragin
All Rights Reserved
First Edition

ISBN: 1-57143-113-6

Library of Congress Catalog Card Number 2004090915

Editors: Kim Klescewski and Richard Harris
Design and Production: Richard Harris
Author Photograph: Nadine Payn

Distributed in Canada by Jaguar Book Group c/o Fraser Direct,
100 Armstrong Way, Georgetown, ON L7G 5S4

Distributed in the United Kingdom and Europe by
Roundhouse Publishing, Ltd., Millstone, Limers Lane, Northam,
North Devon EX39 2RG, United Kingdom

Printed in Canada by Transcontinental Printing

To my Mother and Father

Acknowledgments

This book beat the odds—it was published. Invaluable help came from many people. Tom Tucker, President and CEO of the Council of Compulsive Gambling of California, arranged interviews with compulsive gamblers and supplied me with a myriad of gambling data.

The manuscript was nudged into final form with help from Roger Rapoport, Kim Klescewski, and Richard Harris of RDR Books; David Rompf, Barrie Jean Borich; Laney College English Professors Jerry Herman and Matthew M. Goldstein; and Laney Librarian Evelyn Lord. A bolt of confidence was provided to me by Virgina Conover, creative writing teacher at Louis Pasteur Jr. High School in Los Angeles, circa 1953.

Pathological gambling researchers were generous with their time. Sound advice and guidance came from Dr. Richard J. Rosenthal, Dr. Paul Good, Dr. Seth Eisen, Dr. David Comings, Professor Richard E. Vatz, and Professor Earl L. Grinols.

Thanks to Keith Whyte of the National Council on Problem Gambling, Felix Solomon, Dennis Kuby, Rochelle Caper, Bill Dragin and Ruthe Abel.

Thanks to my weekly "poker therapy" group—Marty, Randy, Norm, Tom (aka New Guy), Stan, Larry, Charles, Ken H., Ken S., Moses, Rob, and David.

A special appreciation to all the compulsive gamblers who confided in me.

And finally, profound gratitude to Dr. Nadine Michele Payn, a wife with immeasurable patience, superb editing skills and psychological insight. And a special thank you to Ana Maria Dragin, our daughter, a teenager blessed with talent—and tolerance for a workaholic father.

Contents

Part I

MY ROLE MODEL

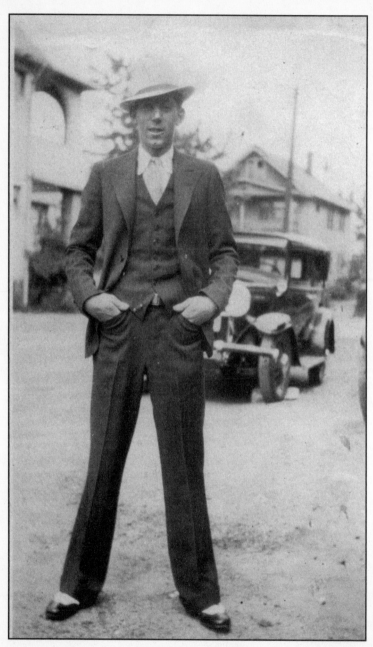

Phil Dragin, around 1932

Chapter 1

Impulse Control Disorder

There's no such thing as a lucky gambler. There are just winners and losers. The winners are those who control the game—all the rest are suckers.

—Meyer Lansky

STEVE WYNN AND I HAVE A FEW THINGS IN COMMON. Family values, for instance. Born the same year, we both visited Las Vegas as children with our gambling-addicted fathers. Wynn became a billionaire Las Vegas impresario, and I helped make him rich. Wynn soon learned that "if you want to make money in a casino, the answer is to own one." I was simply seduced. For decades I would battle gambling addiction while Wynn and his ilk pocketed billions. And I'd do it again. Pluck me from this century and deposit me in the fresh neon of the Flamingo Hotel of the 1950s and I'd swoon once more. Toss in the glitz and glamour, sex and alcohol—and those greenbacks waiting to be picked—and I'd continue the lifelong love affair.

There's no mystery about those who, like Wynn, are inclined toward owning "the house." It's guaranteed gravy. You walk around with a frozen smile and watch the suckers crushed by the immutable odds.

But what's my excuse? I have no shortage of people to blame, but no one put a gun to my head and forced me to toss those dice across the green felt again and again. No one arranged my nights of grinding insomnia as I replayed every bad bet, relived every moment of anguish.

Somewhere, somehow my gambling obsession turned into an obsession with gamblers—the good, the bad, and (especially) the addicted. Why do rational people continue to touch the flame?

During one glorious spurt I took myself out of action and devoured everything I could find on gambling addiction. Doing so produced a modified gambling high. Then I interviewed compulsive gamblers to fit theory with flesh. My father, of course, got microscopic treatment. The result is this book, my odyssey of discovery. What follows is my fitful story, peopled with desperate but hopeful souls.

Working on this book, I felt a special affinity with the late Damon Runyon, a fellow journalist who shared my fascination with gambling and gamblers. A master of the happy ending, Runyon created New Yawk gangsters who exuded warmth and likability. Their revolvers were transformed by his typewriter into "betsies," and people were not murdered but "croaked." This book's title comes from a Runyon short story called "A Nice Price," in which a character called Sam the Gonoph observes, "I long ago come to the conclusion that all life is 6–5 against." Who can argue?

Runyon (1884–1946) did not live to see his short stories transformed into the smash Broadway musical *Guys and Dolls* (1950), immortalizing such characters as Nathan Detroit, Sky Masterson and the scratchy-voiced Adelaide. The Frank Loesser musical would be revived in 1992 starring Nathan Lane as his namesake, Nathan Detroit, and what are the odds of that?

Still later, in 2002, I observed the Runyon legacy on The Strip in Las Vegas. A slow stroll at dusk from The Mirage to Hotel Paris took me past Steve Wynn's stately Bellagio Hotel. As the shimmering lake gave way to arching water spouts, I stood among the thick crowd as the disembodied voice of Frank Sinatra rang out with "Luck Be a Lady," the Sky Masterson tour de force from *Guys and Dolls*.

I was transfixed. Most of the throng was blissfully unaware that the singer had long since departed this world. Or that this multi-laned strip was once a dusty two-lane road with perhaps three hotels. They were in the ultimate Fantasyland.

Perhaps Damon Runyon's glamorous, fantastical world represents the winning streak, when you might as well be in some perfectly scored musical. (New York New York hotel in Las Vegas would be the perfect setting.) Then comes reality in the form of the nasty house edge. What really matters, the voice of experience shouts, is where you are at the end of the game. And aren't we all bucking 6-to-5 odds?

We gamblers are rational in most ways. But put us under the casino's neon blaze, and we melt like the Wicked Witch of the West. Psychiatrists say we have an "impulse control disorder." Even Congress took up our plight, creating the National Gambling Impact Study Commission. The commission spent three years amassing data, then issued a slick, voluminous report in 1999 spiked with red flags:

> Over the past 25 years, the United States has been transformed from a nation in which legalized gambling was a limited and a relatively rare phenomenon into one in which such activity is common and growing. . . As gambling sites proliferate on the Internet and telephone gambling is legalized in more states, an increasingly large fraction of the public can place a bet without ever leaving home at all. Universally available, 'round-the-clock gambling may soon be a reality."

It's already a reality. The commission's dire warnings about "pathological gambling" and a suggested "pause in gambling expansion" have been passed over like roadkill. Witness Indian casinos' unchecked building boom. The "gaming industry" reaps billions per year, fortified with lobbyists whose patrons despise risk.

Here's blunt testimony to our national obsession: "In the single year of 2001, 51 million Americans—more than a quarter of the population over age

21—visited a casino, chalking up a national total of almost 300 million visits," writes Marc Cooper in *The Nation*. "More than 430 commercial casinos nationwide brought in $26.5 billion in revenue—two and a half times what Americans spent on movie tickets, $5 billion more than they spent on DVDs and videos, and $3 billion more than on cosmetics and toiletries." Some casino patrons gamble for entertainment. Others have less healthy reasons. Gambling industry officials say that compulsive and problem gamblers account for fewer than two percent; anti-gambling sources say it's between 10 and 20 percent.

Newspapers print daily point spreads. Super Bowl gambling tops $5 billion in a one-day orgy of wagering. Even the war in Iraq drew more than $1 million in illegal wagers on the Internet. One of many betting options was the fate of Saddam Hussein by June 30, 2003: (1) Still president of Iraq and in control of Baghdad, 2:1. (2) Captured by the US, 2:1. (3) Dead, 3:2. (4) Missing in action, 7:4. And (5) in political exile, 2:1.

I have no desire to shut down casinos, although I have empathy for those so engaged. Rather, I would like to see the gambling industry invest huge sums in education to help prevent addiction. Otherwise, as one of my compulsive gambling subjects suggests, "ten years down the road gambling will be where tobacco is now." Can't you picture Las Vegas/Atlantic City impresario Steve Wynn and his brethren appearing in Congress, arms raised in oath about "the myth" of gambling addiction? Millions of Americans can already attest to the consequences of gambling. I've yet to encounter anyone who doesn't know someone with a gambling problem.

Who keeps the gambling industry flourishing? Surely I've done my share, having signed on with that cadre of dreamers, a group determined to overturn the iron law of probability. I'd find myself swiping my ATM card "just one more time" at the casino, betting my last two bucks at the track, or leaving the card club at 5 a.m. broke, bleary-eyed, and disgusted. I have managed to avoid prison, bankruptcy, psychosis, and having my knees cracked by thugs. Still, I paid. But even the most punch-drunk boxer eventually peers through the haze and wonders why. Do I want to climb back in the ring, or take a moment to count my remaining brain cells?

Chapter 2

Highbrow Deception

The next best thing to playing and winning is playing and losing. The main thing is to play. —Nick the Greek (Dandalos)

Gambling is suicide without death. —André Malraux

THESE TWO QUOTES HAUNT THE COMPULSIVE GAMBLER. I've embraced both concepts. I've thrilled to filling an inside straight and watching a mountain of chips shoved my way. And I've tossed the dice across the green felt and watched them ricochet off the back wall, dance crazily, and land on the hard ten, eliciting screams, massive payoffs, and group elation. And I'm the hero!

But I've also marched trancelike through the casino after uncontrollable losses with my insides on fire, barely containing myself, treading lightly so as not to explode. So when The Greek says "the next best thing is gambling and losing," I respectfully demur. Gambling and losing, for the addict, is hell. Some of the best fiction is written in the head of the compulsive gambler; it's his rationale for staying "in action"—an odds-on shot at self-destruction.

I don't mean to denigrate The Greek (1883-1966), whose name was spoken with reverence in our home. His legendary status was never in question. In his book *Gambling Secrets of Nick the Greek*, Ted Thackrey, Jr. writes:

7

During the 60 years of his career, he estimated that he had won and lost more than $500,000,000; gone from rags to riches and back to rags again 73 separate times; and on one occasion actually had time to count and be astounded by a single winning score of $50,000,000.

The Greek was an icon of immense proportion; he never lacked for backers when his cash was depleted. But few problem gamblers today have that luxury. They must replenish their stake by any means necessary.

My own rationale for gambling was highbrow deception. I had glommed onto Herman Melville's *Moby Dick* character Ishmael and the famous doldrums that sent him packing: "Whenever I find myself growing grim about the mouth," Ishmael says, "whenever it is a dark, drizzly November in my soul . . . then, I account it high time to get to sea as soon as I can."

Ishmael sought release in the "watery part of the world." I sought it at the green felt of the crap table. As I approached the casino, the Las Vegas Strip, Reno or Atlantic City, I shared Ishmael's lust for adventure and the heady thrill of total risk. For me the great white whale was hot dice and the lucky blackjack deck. I was hooked.

Where better to fight the eternal battle than here in the casino: clockless, windowless, with blazing neon, thinly clad cocktail waitresses, clanging slot machines, and one's fortitude enhanced by an unending supply of free alcohol? In fact, if it weren't for the house edge guaranteed to grind players into submission, this would be a plausible escape.

Compulsives know too well what time it is. You see them hovering around the ATM at five minutes to midnight. A new day: those with a daily limit can squeeze out a few more crisp hundreds, transform them into chips, and chase the dream a while longer. Some will return after the 24-hour cycle, dazed, half-delirious, determined to "get even."

But then deep in the throes of my addiction I took a tentative step out of quicksand. Leaving a Nevada casino after a monster loss, with a headache fueled by rage, I slammed the car door against a pristine, snowy evening and headed south from Reno into California. A pitched battle throbbed in my brain. Why couldn't I stop? I was $1,500 ahead. Why keep gambling? Why subject myself to this? Ten minutes later I was plotting my return trip. Next time I'd leave a winner. Next time! If I'm $1,500 ahead, I assure myself, I'll put away $1,000 and play out the $500. Then leave.

But I've heard this tune before. After blowing the $500, I rationalize that $900 is a pretty good score, so I play out $100. And another $100. And another. But would there be a next time? Or had my quest begun? Did I really seek answers? Or did I truly prefer the delicious mental fog of the casino? I blared the stereo, opened the window and inhaled the chill. Was this epiphany . . . or delusion? And if I did want to understand gambling's tenacious hold—let's say I really did—where would I start?

As the car moved through swirling snow, I contemplated the challenge—time subtracted from gambling to pursue the question of . . . why gamble? My mind wrestled with the paradox. There was clearly an urge to get back to the casino . . . and yet a seed of curiosity about addiction fought for a hearing. So the drive south turned into an internal courtroom battle. I was both defense and prosecution. As the defense attorney, I shut up and allowed the prosecution a chance to cite the benefits of a quest for the gambling demon. Would such a quest supplant my gambling urge? No answer. And if I faced off against the demon, would that change anything? Again, no answer. Casino images—neon and noise, sex and alcohol—made fitful appearances.

Yet curiosity wielded a power of its own. Contemplating the quest, I knew my first step had to be research. As a journalist I had unearthed data for stories on everything from alcoholic pilots to pet wolves. I had even taken a graduate school class in journalism research methods. The secret for the quest, I knew, was to transfer the gambling passion to a passion for discovery. If the casino should overpower me, that in itself would be a lesson. I'd scotch the venture and give in to gambling fever.

Predating the Vegas casino, I was about to learn, lay centuries of gambling addiction tales. Even Aristotle, Einstein and Gandhi would weigh in before I was done. I'd track down history's first mention of compulsive gamblers and trace the long tradition of gambling cheats, wastrels and reformers. I'd return to the days when crooked gamblers, called "gamesters" or "sharpers," prospered—except when vigilantes became judge, jury and executioner. I'd run across legends like "Titanic Thompson," so named because he gambled every last dollar, and when he lost he sank like his namesake. It's a lush history, peopled with riverboat dandies, politicos on the take, and three-card monte crooks who'd bilk their own grandmothers. I'd imbibe these historical gems along the way as I scoped out my main quarry:

Why do some gamblers become addicted?

What about Gamblers Anonymous, I wondered. Group fixes never appealed to me, but I'd find out. Compulsive gamblers in recovery are eager to talk, sharing stories of pain and loss. I'd also question today's leading researchers in gambling addiction—like the expert who suggested two key questions to ask my compulsive gambling subjects:

"How did you feel when you first crossed the line of deception to cover up gambling losses?"

"As a child, what importance did your family place on money?"

I knew exactly where to start my quest . . .

Chapter 3

What Good Is Money?

The gambler is apparently the last optimist; he is a creature totally unmoved by experience.
—Dr. Edmund Bergler in *The Psychology of Gambling* (1958)

MY FATHER GLIMPSED THE MAGNIFICENT YELLOW STUTZ BEARCAT CONVERTIBLE and went into rapture. At the wheel was Johnny Scalish wearing the uniform of his trade: pinstriped suit, vest, watch fob, roll collar, fedora tilted rakishly, and gleaming black leather shoes. Scalish was a gangster on the move. He would rule the Cleveland Mafia from 1944 until his death in 1976. But this particular day was in the late 1920s. My father, rail-thin with an attitude, was in his teens. His admiration for Scalish was boundless. My father was torn between two worlds. Would he choose the stylish gangster's life or hook up with the gorgeous brunette he'd been dating and settle down to a responsible life?

"What good is money?" my father often said. "It makes most people miserable." He said it with finality. With an edge. Sometimes he'd say it as a pre-emptive strike to ward off an argument about the money he had just lost. The position was unassailable. Yet it was wholly contradictory.

My father craved riches. Early on, he fancied himself George Raft, the gangster-cum-Hollywood leading man. How my father might reach that

11

pinnacle was anyone's guess. But logic would not play a part. Logic says you go broke, you live on the streets. You strike it rich, you go first class.

My father went broke and moved to Beverly Hills. True, it was a one-room apartment with no amenities, but he was near his club, where in palmier days he had acquired a lifetime membership. Now he would kibitz with the likes of actors Peter Falk and Paul Newman—with no income of his own to speak of. How did my father manage basic survival, let alone frequent the ritzy box seats at Hollywood Park racetrack?

Now in his eighties, my father eagerly recalls a life of nonstop gambling action and regret. He sits for my interviews while the TV silently blazes the day's sporting events. "I always had friends that would come through," he tells me. "We're going to the track and they'd say, 'Here's five hundred, I know you're broke.' I'd say I don't know when I can pay it back and they'd say 'Do I look worried?' So I took it. What could I do?"

It would be a simple matter to paint my father in Runyonesque terms, a world-class schmoozer of immense charm whose gambling passion wouldn't cease. I could toss in that he quit high school at 16 and consorted with gangsters in Cleveland. But it would be a hatchet job of singular dimension. Besides, when he related the following gambling anecdote to me, decades after the fact, I recoiled with that cold shiver reserved for those about whom we care deeply.

During his short-lived Beverly Hills period, he recalls, "a guy who knew a guy from the club asked if I was looking for some action." Sure, my father tells him. The guy gives my father a phone number and a code. My father calls, gets the Beverly Hills address and shows up. "It's a casino, right in the living room," my father says. "Plush." Ten minutes later three guys barge in. "The first thing I see is the shotguns," my father says. "I almost shit in my pants." The gunmen scoop up all the cash in the game and rip a Rolex off a limp wrist. "Nice setup," my father says blankly.

I hear this story and I'm bleeding inside. With a slightly different click of fate, my father could have been blown away in a grisly shooting ("Six Gamblers Slain / In Bev Hills Home Casino"). Or worse, my father could have been one of the bad guys.

* * *

It was bad guys of a different era—Cossacks, police and thugs—that drove the Drashinskys from Odessa, Russia. My paternal grandfather was a barrel maker when things started to heat up for the Jews of Odessa as the year 1900 dawned. They called them "pogroms"—a Russian word for devastation. More accurately, the pogroms instigated against the Jews of Odessa were murderous rampages. What was the offense of the Jews? They stood up to the Tsarist empire by helping workers win the right to form unions, improve working conditions and decide their own fate. Centuries-old anti-Semitism was easily stoked, producing the conflagration.

In 1905 there was a genuine revolution of workers in Odessa. The authorities quashed it, of course. But it was a dress rehearsal for the Bolshevik Revolution of 1917. My grandfather didn't stick around to see it. Soon after my father was born in 1912, my grandfather, Aaron Drashinsky, made his way to America. (His cousin had come decades earlier, landing in Cleveland.) Two years later the rest of the family—my grandmother and her six children—made the same arduous voyage. My father was just an infant on the trip.

The family emerged from Ellis Island chaos with the name "Dragin." They spoke Russian and Yiddish in their new Cleveland home. But my father, the youngest child, would have none of this foreign stigma. He was the family's self-appointed emissary to the street—a marvelous mix of pickup baseball games, crap games, poker games, hanging out at the schoolyard until dusk, and coed outings in rakish convertibles as the Twenties roared to a close.

My father's recounting of his past is suffused with two themes: First, no one in the family showed him "what was what." This included dental hygiene, diet, and the importance of school. (It's tempting to wonder how his siblings got the word.) Second, his praise for Fannie, my mother, known as Fae after adolescence, is unstinting. "Without her," he says, "I'd have wound up on skid row."

* * *

Cleveland's Palace Theatre featured top vaudevillians of the day. My father made it into the Palace, through the stage door no less, thanks to a young Cleveland Press reporter. "This guy's a friend of mine and he's on the way over to the Palace and asks if I want to come along," my father says. "I love music, vaudeville, theater—all of it. So I go. I'm introduced to the guy in charge. He says to me, 'Where are you working?' I'm 16 or 17 at the time. 'Nowhere,' I tell him. 'How would you like a job?' he says.

"He wants me to run bets for the performers, who love to play the horses. So I take their bets down the street to the bookie; I have a secret knock to get in. Not big bets, maybe $2 or $5. But running bets for these headliners—Jolson, Cantor, Cab Callaway—was a thrill. A guy makes a score, I get a tip."

My father's eldest brother, Benjamin, was a concert violinist who had studied at the Odessa Conservatory. "Ben hobnobbed with doctors and lawyers," my father recalls. "He called me a bum. Acted like a big shot. He looked down on us. He should have helped me more. He tried to teach me violin but I hated it. He should have told me what was what." Another member of the Dragin household recalled things differently. "Your father wanted nothing to do with the family," she told me. "He had his own crowd. He wanted a glamorous life."

What if the family had not left Odessa? If they had toughed it out under the Tsar and the nascent machinations of Vladimir Lenin? It's hard to picture Pavel Drashinsky in the Odessa schoolroom, dutifully tracing his Cyrillic letters. More likely he'd be on the mean streets, nose bloodied, cussing out his "pure" Russian antagonists.

But he was in America. He'd make the most of it and try not to make the worst of himself. America was the land of chance. The French author Alex de Tocqueville toured the US in the 1830s and then observed in *Democracy in America:*

Those who live in the midst of democratic fluctuations have always before their eyes the image of chance, and they end by liking all undertakings in which chance plays a part.

De Tocqueville got it right. Americans were gamblers all, from the first lottery in 1777 to raise funds for the Revolutionary War right through next year's Super Bowl. Words written by David Pietrusza (in *Rothstein*) about our nation's most notorious gambler, Arnold Rothstein, the man who fixed the 1919 World Series, surely apply to my father:

Risk energized Arnold, made him feel important, provided him with the potential for great riches, and set him apart from the stodgy world of his father. To Arnold Rothstein—and so many of his contemporaries—gambling was modernity. It was America.

But gambling to excess? My father's obsession cannot easily be traced to the "nature vs. nurture" debate. He got little nurturing at home. He was the family's first English speaker, and with that he gravitated toward those he perceived were able to talk their way into anything. Culturally, he qualified for gambling's mystic thrall. Jews and Asians lead the league in the obsession, although no group is counted out.

There's more to it, though. A passion for gambling is often a rejection of the grown-up world of planning, delayed gratification, a full-functioning superego. It's no wonder my father shunned violin lessons. If Pauly could have picked up the delicate instrument and sounded like Heifetz in ten minutes, he might have pursued it. Tossing dice can be learned before the two whirling cubes hit the wall, then bounce back and reveal your fate. A winning toss is spiked by peer-group approval.

So my father rejected the Dragin household with its rich Old World Yiddish culture of extended family, punctuated by music and long meals and political talk. Recounting his days at the schoolyard, my father rhapsodizes: "It was wonderful. Guys would come after work and start a base-ball game. I was just 12 or 13. They were always short a guy so I'd play. Afterward they'd start a crap game. I was their friend, so I'd stand there and watch. They were in their teens and twenties. Seems like I was always with older guys."

Although I've only seen my father shooting dice as an adult, it's not hard to picture him the moment he discovered his passion. A crap game is a rite of passage; the grounded, sensible teenager sees wins and losses as just that. There's no magic. It's as thrilling as accounting principles. When the game's over it's over; it gets no more thought.

But for a kid soon to perceive a hole in his dream of wealth and power, it takes on a deep symbolism. For Pauly, the dice were an extension of his being. When they rang true, it was very personal. He became like a prized athlete on steroids—very powerful. Early on he busted a game and found himself thumbing a wad of green. His brothers might possess musical talent or business savvy, but Pauly had guts and bravado, and some special friends who knew life's shortcuts. Gambling losses were an inconvenience he'd learn to deal with—as would others whose lives were linked to Pauly's.

From the schoolyard my father graduated to Amato's Pool Hall, where he met the sleek mobster Johnny Scalish. The local hoodlums would come into the poolroom, take their guns out of their holsters, and put them under the counter. "You can't shoot pool with guns. We thought nothing of it," my father says in reflective amazement. "The cops all knew my first name."

At this point in the interview my mother saunters over. Incredibly, she still harbors ambivalence about my father's teenage persona. Was she really dating a man whose name was known by the cops? She listens to his remi-niscences with a mixture of pride and regret.

"One time the cops came in and told the gangsters to line up against the wall," my father continues. "So we—two Italian guys and me—we lined up against the wall, too."

My mother laughs an I-should-have-had-my-head-examined laugh. But the nostalgia is too rich to ignore; she also is transported to Cleveland and the passion of youth—a hint of glamour still visible beneath the loose skin and battle weary visage. Had I a magic wand, I'd exorcise her every remnant of regret.

My father himself narrowly missed prison when he was nudged out of a threesome plotting a gas station stickup. "They got caught," my father says. "Cops grabbed 'em. Luckily, I got out."

My father stiffens in his chair, proceeding with his unscheduled confessional. "One time," he says, "I saw a guy get shot. Right in the street. Dropped. Just like that. I turned and didn't go up that street. I'd been told that if I ever see something like that, don't mix in."

Perhaps the most memorable sight at Amato's Pool Hall was the squirrely little guy who strode in one afternoon desperate for cash. "He says he needs $500 to bet on a horse, a sure thing," my father recalls. "There're all these Italian guys standing around. This guy says his name is Mickey Cohen and he's 'in' with mobsters. He's pleading for money. But no dice. No one's ever heard of him. Now Mickey's getting mad. Finally Tony Galotti—very tough guy—says he'll loan him the $500 until tomorrow. And that's the last we see of Mickey Cohen. The horse lost. And Tony's saying how he'll 'take care' of Mickey one day. No one had any doubts what he meant."

My father would cross Cohen's path years later in Los Angeles. Cohen had achieved major hoodlum status in LA, with a front as a haberdasher. He had his own take on violence and a vague moral code: "I've done a lot of things in my day," Cohen writes in *Mickey Cohen: In My Own Words*. "But I never killed just for killing."

My father was more inclined toward presenting the image of a gangster than being an actual gangster. One photo shows him around age 20, posed like a George Raft stand-in—three piece suit, wide-brimmed hat, two-toned shoes, hands in pockets over immaculate creases down each pant leg. His legs are spread in a stance of mild rebellion, his lips starting to form a smile but in truth concealing bad teeth.

Driving Scalish and his pals around town—they were partial to James Cagney movies—in the gaudy yellow convertible was heaven for my father. "Once Scalish drove up to the poolroom and told me to go pick up his girlfriend Rosalyn and bring her back," my father recalls. Turned out Rosalyn lived one gravel driveway from the Dragin family home. "I tooted the horn for Rosalyn and my father stuck his head out the window and saw me," my father says, cringing 70 years after the fact. "He knew it was a gangster's car. Boy, I caught hell that night."

My father met my mother in Hollywood script fashion. "I had just bought this Lyon-Taylor suit for $27," he recalls. "And a few of us guys went to this party on Union Avenue. We weren't actually invited." The host blocked the door. "Let's crash it," my father said. Once inside, he looked around "to see who I could see" and there was Fannie. "Oh my God," my father said. "Who is that?" It didn't take him long to find out. And he quickly told his friend Sam: "This is it. I'm going to marry this girl."

The raucous 1920s ended abruptly with the stock market crash. Enter the thirties, a miserable post-party hangover. When the stock market crashed in 1929, my father was 17. His brother Ben, however, lost a regal sum in the collapse of the market. My father's challenge was not so much with keeping a job as keeping his paycheck. "I was always in hock," he says. "Guys would loan me money. That was the problem."

Half a century later, my mother still disputes that claim. "The problem with your father," she says, "was that he loved to gamble. And noth-ing—or no one—was going to stop him." This was not an after-the-fact revelation. Says my mother: "Early in our marriage your father's boss's wife took me aside at a family gathering. She said she couldn't take it anymore. She called me into the bathroom and asked if I knew what Phil (no longer

"Pauly") was doing all day Saturday. 'He said he was working, but he was really gambling,' she told me."

Worse, my mother learned, my father would borrow enough to make it look like he had been paid. He threatened to take off and never come back if the relatives didn't lend him the money. "That night at home we had a big fight," my mother recalled. "He promised never to do it again."

Like most compulsive gamblers, my father made convincing promises.

It was gambling joints like Moe Dalitz's Harvard Club on Cleveland's south side that drew my father like a drunk to schnapps.

"Harvard Club was the classy place," my father says. "Guys wore tuxes. They'd line up at a corner downtown and Dalitz would send cars to pick them up and drive them to the club, which was just outside the Cleveland city limits. It was all illegal, of course. Someone got paid off."

My father himself frequented the less stylish Thomas Club. "It was like a barn. Sawdust on the floor. About four or five crap tables. No chips. They used silver dollars."

Dalitz, who had an alliance with Meyer Lansky, would later front the funds to build the Desert Inn Hotel in Vegas and buy into several other hotels. Investigative reporters Sally Denton and Roger Morris write in *The Money and the Power: The Making of Las Vegas and Its Hold on America, 1947–2000*:

In 1950, visitors to Wilbur Clark's luxurious new Desert Inn might see Clark moving affably from table to table, or even one of his more famous and frequent guests, J. Edgar Hoover, crossing the lobby. What they could not see was that the controlling owner, Moe Dalitz—known as the toughest Jewish mobster in Vegas—had once killed a Cleveland city councilman who stood in his way, carried a long history of what one writer called ruthless beatings, unsolved murders and shakedowns, had bribed his way to the big fix, as two reporters described it, in a half-dozen city halls around the nation, and now presided over the skim of millions a year for Lansky, the Cleveland mob, and his other secret partners.

It would be two decades before my father would patronize Dalitz's Nevada establishments—the start of my father's second tier of serious gambling. Until then, he was content to gamble away his paycheck and borrow money.

What if my father had crossed paths with Dalitz in those days? Both men were ambitious and charming. They could have been fast friends. It's an intriguing "what if . . ." My father could easily have yielded up his future to the mob, convinced he could be a player without blood on his hands. Of course he couldn't, but if he had tried I'd have wound up one of those kids ignoring the brutality and praising dad for "always being a good father." I've heard more than once how these mobsters' kids cling to such familial rationales.

In one of his many truck driving jobs, my father was shouted down from his cab by some mob types in a Cadillac. "You a union guy?" my father was asked. He was not. "Then you can't drive." These were bulky bosses of the International Brotherhood of Teamsters, flexing their new muscle. (Thirty years down the road, the Teamsters' pension fund would be illegally poured into Vegas expansion.)

Dismayed and out of work, my father took it up with his pal John Scalish. Nothing could be done. "We don't get along too good with those guys," Scalish told him. But Scalish had a relative who knew someone who knew someone who set my father up with a union truck driving job.

My father's gambling habit apparently was not enough to undo his relationship with my mother, who, like him, lived at home. She longed to attend college, but family obligations came first. She worked in the little family grocery store on Union Avenue.

"It was the depth of the Depression," she recalled. "No one had money. People got charity. We'd write down what they bought, and how much, and send the bill off to some government agency. Eventually, we'd get a check." My mother recalled going off to school with a salami sandwich and strawberry pop made at the store. Instead of college, she found herself working at Bamberger-Rhine Fall Knit Goods—for $8 per week.

What was her attraction to the sleek guy whose future spelled disaster? "I wish I knew," my mother says after sixty-five years of marriage. "We just got paired off. We were together. That was it."

They were both blessed with movie-star good looks. This may have been The Great Depression, but my parents seemed to find sustenance in old fashioned romance. They even had their song—"Star Dust" by Hoagy Carmichael.

My parents have boxes of tattered black-and-white snapshots. One shows the couple seated on park bleachers, my father a step above my mother, his hands resting tenderly on her shoulders. The scene is magical. After dusk there's bound to be a brilliant yellow Harvest moon and fireflies flitting about. "Mystics Outing, Aug. 3, 1930," is scrawled atop the photo in thin blue ink.

A few years later, August 13, 1933, they would marry, putting the kibosh on my father's days at Amato's Pool Hall and palling around with mobsters. Said my father: "That ended that." Now he was the 21-year-old breadwinner. It must have pained him that the very year he got married Prohibition was repealed and the mob activities shifted from rum running to gambling. In Cleveland alone, yearly profits from the numbers game ran as high as $10 million. Surely my father could have been a well-paid cog in the illegal gambling industry, far less dangerous than transporting illegal booze.

My father's own destructive gambling, however, continued. Did he ever analyze it? "It was different in those days," he says, ignoring the question. "You had to worry about crooked dice. These days, they're happy if you win a couple grand. They [as in Vegas] know you'll be back."

This pattern of my father answering the "how" rather than the "why" of his own gambling never ceased. Yet I could not condemn him for his destructive habit, for gambling—the psychological need for suffusing oneself in risk—would course through my blood, too.

Chapter 4

"Seriously Disturbed and Regressed"

Everyone reaches out for risk. Everyone craves it. Some people may unconsciously seek out dangerous personal relationships. Rather than settle on a stable romance, they create an explosive situation in which they stalk a difficult reward while risking great pain. They are gamblers in the act of gambling. —Mike Caro

MY INITIAL FORAY INTO THE LITERATURE ABOUT GAMBLING FELT ODD; I SOUGHT answers to questions that I'm not sure I really wanted answered. Yet the research produced a rush—not the scintillating rush of Vegas neon and the riffle of the blackjack deck, but nonetheless, something stirred within me. Was it because, as with the bouncing dice, I wasn't sure of the result? Would I identify with gamblers I'd interview? Place myself in "recovery"? Join GA? Or would the entire quest prove salutary, a welcome respite from the tyranny of the house edge?

Knowing full well that gambling theories of such heavy hitters as Sigmund Freud might be outdated, I pursued my odyssey into rumblings of the unconscious mind.

I began with an article by Robert Linder ("The Psychodynamics of Gambling," 1950), who reviewed the theories of prominent psychoanalysts of the early 20th century. Ernst Simmel (1920) viewed the gambler as "seriously disturbed and regressed." What Simmel meant (a psychologist explained to me) is that in early childhood infants and toddlers long for food, love and attention, known in psychoanalytic jargon as "narcissistic supplies." He posited that gamblers were denied these comforts by their parents; therefore, gambling is a repeated effort to get fundamental human needs fulfilled. Unfortunately, gamblers are now adults who use, according to Simmel, "primitive techniques" in a "hopeless reversion to outmoded and unsuitable modes of behavior and thought."

(Perhaps some Las Vegas entrepreneur could exploit the theory by building a theme hotel called The Neon Nursery. The possibilities are endless: slot machines with rattles; pink and blue walls; cocktail waitresses replaced by nursemaids serving warm milk. The high rollers would have their own area—the Womb Room.)

Freud (1929) challenged Simmel with a new appraisal of what motivates gamblers. In an essay ostensibly about Dostoyevsky and patricide, the father of psychoanalysis related the pathological compulsion to gamble to what he saw as the pervasive conflict over masturbation. In fact, Freud believed that the compulsive gambler was so racked with guilt over masturbation that he was compelled to find a subconscious substitute. This reductionism may cause a contemporary reader to chuckle.

Theodore Reik (1940) put a slightly different spin on Freud's theory, recognizing gambling "as a modern form of oracle through which the gambler seeks to penetrate the future and thereby to obtain an answer to the question that unconsciously plagues him: Will I be punished or forgiven for my trespasses (masturbation)? Destiny, 'the ultimate father surrogate,' is thus besought for an answer through the vicissitudes of the play and its chance-determined outcome."

It was not Freud but Dr. Edmund Bergler who, in 1958, wrote the century's definitive book on compulsive gambling, *The Psychology of Gambling*. Its purpose was "to substantiate, with clinical proof, the theory that the gambler has an unconscious wish to lose—and therefore always loses in the long run." (This would be a tough sell to today's desperate gambling addict who had just lost his bankroll, maxed out his credit cards, and is contemplating the view from the casino-hotel's 40th floor.)

Gathering his data from case studies of his own patients, Bergler concluded, "The gambler is apparently the last optimist. He is a creature totally unmoved by experience." Many of Bergler's findings about gambling addiction would be cited by medical experts for decades to come. Central to his theory about problem gamblers is that "the game precludes all other interests." Bergler writes:

> The mental energy of the pathologic gambler is almost constantly concentrated on gambling, on computing chances and making prognostications. His fantasies and daydreams center around this one idea; the pathological concentration overshadows everything else—vocation, love, hobbies . . . Every gambler gives the impression of a man who has signed a contract with Fate, stipulating that persistence must be rewarded.

This I could easily validate; during my gambling mania, my mind constantly drifted back to disastrous play at a recent gambling session and forward to my next chance for redemption.

Bergler says that the more intelligent gambler "stresses the irrational motive in gambling: the thrill component." Bergler documents the "thrill" by citing a letter written by Dostoyevsky: "The main point is the game itself. On my oath, it is not greed for money, despite the fact that I need money badly."

That notion of the game being everything rings out through history. In a variant that predated Nick the Greek, Lord Byron (1788-1824) wrote:

> In play there are two pleasures for your choosing
> The one is winning, and the other is losing.

Further, Bergler says of gambling:

> It is a dangerous neurosis. The gambler doesn't gamble because he consciously decides to gamble; he is propelled by unconscious

forces over which he has no control. He is an objectively sick person who is subjectively unaware that he is sick.

It is at this point that most problem gamblers turn a deaf ear. Mention "the unconscious" and they want no part of your theory. But Bergler is worth pursuing. "The best approach to the problem of the gambler's unconscious psychology," he writes, "is to examine his illogical, senseless certainty that he will win."

Bergler traces that certainty to childhood and its "fiction of omnipotence." Bergler cites Freud's conclusion that childhood is a time of overinflated ego and belief that reality can be controlled by whim. Contemporary theorists call this "magical thinking." But it can't last. Bergler writes: "Real experience gradually destroys this fiction, an experience which is probably the deepest disappointment of childhood."

In short, for a child to become an adult, he must face reality and learn to acknowledge immutable laws over which he has no control. He doesn't fight battles he cannot win. The adult saves his energy for "real" adversaries.

Bergler concedes that as adults we retain a tiny part of the childhood fiction that we can get what we want simply because we want it. But normally reality has a leavening effect on the healthy adult. However, continues Bergler, there is "one exceptional situation in life" when reality is discarded in favor of childhood grandiosity. "That is gambling. There blind chance rules, chance which in games of 'pure' gambling cannot be influenced by logic or intelligence."

For a more ego-shattering theory of the gambler-as-child, consider Maurice Maeterlinck (1862-1949):

There is a great deal of puerile vanity about the gambler. Taken all in all, he is a child still seeking his place in the universe. He has not yet realized his position. He thinks himself peerless in the face of destiny. In his self-infatuation he expects the unknown or unknowable to do for him what it does not do for anyone whomsoever.

And he expects this for no reason, simply because he is himself and because others have not that privilege. He must tempt fate incessantly, hurriedly, anxiously, in I know not what idle and pretentious hope of learning to know himself from without. Whatever fortune's decision may be, he will find cause for preening himself. If he have no luck, he will feel flattered because he is specially persecuted by fortune; if he be lucky, he will think all the more highly of himself because of the exceptional gifts which she bestows upon him."

To say that problem gamblers revert to the world of childhood where all wishes are granted is a gross oversimplification. But as an "action gambler," I can attest to that uncanny feeling that I'm about to win as I toss the dice across the green felt and my fellow bettors cheer me on. And then I throw the hard ten for payoffs around the board (except for those snakes who bet with the house) and it's high-fives and raucous shouts, and the plunger next to me who wins $2,000 whispers "God Damn, this is better than sex" and I have no argument.

But when I leave the casino hours later, broke, with an ache in my heart, I'm pummeling my psyche. "Of course," Bergler would say. "It's called psychic masochism."

Here's where Bergler gets down and dirty (if not obtuse), but his ideas seem always to lead to revelation: "Gambling unconsciously revives . . . the old childish fantasy of grandeur and megalomania . . . it activates the latent rebellion against logic, intelligence, moderation, morality, and renunciation."

The purveyors of these virtues, according to Bergler, are parents and other authority figures. The gambler's rebellion against them takes the form of regressing to the childhood state of omnipotence in which the laws of logic and probability are defied. ("You're going to do what I command, roulette wheel!") Bergler says that the aggression necessary to rebel activates "a profound unconscious feeling of guilt." He is emphatic that this guilt is completely outside the gambler's awareness. Therefore, *uncon-*

sciously the gambler must punish himself for his aggression. What better punishment than to lose at the very thing he loves?

Bergler goes further. He says the gambler's unconscious wish to lose fuels his motivation to keep on wagering, and he labels this process "psychic masochism." In layperson's terms this means the gambler develops a kind of pleasure in self-pity and righteous indignation (as in "the dice turned cold on me"). Result: you have a "viscious, and endless, circle" of addiction.

Most compulsive (and problem) gamblers would scoff at Bergler and consider his writings "psychobabble." But what's their own explanation for devastating losses? (This is explained in PROFILES.) My father, I'm sure, would have had none of Bergler's theory. My father craved action, and any probing analysis of "why gambling?" would have meant a pause in his frenetic life.

Chapter 5

An Enchanting Witchery

Life itself loses in interest when the highest stakes in the game of living,
life itself, may not be risked. —Sigmund Freud

LAS VEGAS MAY SEEM THE APOGEE OF OUR GAMBLING NATION. But in earlier centuries, Americans were wagering at a frantic pace. "Gamesters"—thieves with a decided edge over the player—presided over the action. Colonists were warned about such scam artists, along with the intrinsic evil and sickness of gambling itself.

Charles Cotton penned *The Compleat Gamester* in 1674, with the cumbersome subtitle: *Or instructions (on) how to play at billiards, trucks, bowls, and chess, together with all manner of useful and most gentile (sic) games either on cards or dice. To which is added, the arts and mysteries of riding, racing, archery, and cock-fighting.*

Besides his sage advice on how to win, Cotton paints an indelible, though hyperbolic, picture of the ill effects of gambling. He writes,

Gaming is an enchanting witchery, gotten betwixt idleness and avarice: An itching disease, that makes some scratch the head, whilst

28

others, as if they were bitten by a tarantula, are laughing themselves to death: Or lastly, it is a paralytic distemper, which seizing the arm of the man cannot choose but shake his elbow.

It hath this ill property above all other vices, that it renders a man incapable of prosecuting any serious action, and makes him always unsatisfied with his own condition; he is either lifted up to the top of mad joy with success, or plung'd to the bottom of despair by misfortune, always in extremes, always in a storm.

Cotton continues in this vein for several more pages, finally concluding of the gambler that "either winning or losing he can never rest satisfied, if he wins he thinks to win more, if he loses he hopes to recover." The book found a welcome reception in the new colonies, for along with those seeking religious freedom others were "gamesters" seeking suckers to bilk. And has it ever been otherwise? Gambling thrived in the colonies despite protests by Puritans and Quakers and "Blue Laws" devised by William Penn.

The French and Spanish left a legacy of gambling games in the early 1800s that would find a welcome home on the Mississippi River and then westward with the Gold Rush of 1849. The most popular was the board game Faro, "the medium of the first extensive cheating at cards ever seen in the United States, and the rock upon which were reared the elaborate gambling houses of the early and middle nineteenth century," writes Herbert Asbury in *Sucker's Progress: An Informal History of Gambling in America from the Colonies to Canfield.*

Craps and roulette also found their entrance to America through New Orleans, although the former was an adaptation of the English game Hazard. Lesser known games such as All Fours, Seven-Up, Pitch, Chuck-a-Luck, Whist and Three-Card Monte were also played during this period—all imports. The only game with a purely American pedigree is Thimble-Rig, a variation of Three-Card Monte, better known as the "Shell Game," wherein the "mark" has to guess which of the three shells has the pea under it. In all cases—unless the bettor was a confederate—the pea was between the middle and index finger of the Thimble Rig tosser.

Cheating was so popular a business that the professional gambler "bought his marked cards, crooked dealing boxes, loaded dice and other apparatus for cheating, all known by the generic name of 'Advantage Tools,' from manufacturers and dealers who advertised openly in the newspapers and circulars sent through the mails," Asbury writes.

One Eastern dealer sent a form letter to each inquiry about his products:

Dear Sir—In reply to yours, there is only one sure way to win at cards, etc., and that is to get Tools to work with and then to use them with discretion, which is the secret of all Gambling and the way that all Gamblers make their money.

The sharpers—known also during the era as "blacklegs"—rarely worked alone, although they often appeared to. A confederate was known as a "capper." He'd win enough to entice a bystander to risk his cash. Naturally, the sharpers had their own language, and a colorful lexicon it was. The following were compiled by Thomas L. Clark in *Cheating Terms in Cards and Dice:*

Bleeder Operator or manager of a gambling establishment who worries that a winning player may leave soon and therefore orders that the player be cheated.

Breastworks Metal contrivance worn under a shirt, vest or jacket for holding a card or cards until needed.

Bust-out joint (1) Illegal gaming establishment. (2) Gaming house specializing in cheating.

Cheese-eater Informer on a cheater in the game or house.

Cold deck Prearranged pack of cards slipped into the game.

Dump-over shot Any of a variety of trick rolls in which the dice land with a predetermined number of pips showing.

Flat-joint Establishment catering to cheaters and crooked gamblers, especially where dice are used.

Floats Dice which have been hollowed out to make one side lighter (detectable by placing in a glass of water).

Greek bottom Second card from the bottom of the deck.

Greek shot Controlled cast of the dice in which both dice hit the backboard, but only one die rolls away.

Hand-mucker Cheater who is adept at sleight of hand; one who easily palms cards.

Hemingway Cheater often at card games. Used as a code word among cheaters to recognize one another.

Jack stripper Jack (usually of spades) shaved slightly to force a cut or allow a confederate to cut the pack from a designated point.

Juice joint Gambling house that uses electricity to control magnetized dice.

Luminous readers Cards marked with a special dye that can be detected only by wearing pink-tinted glasses.

Mechanic One skilled at manipulating cards or dice for cheating.

Pipe salesman Honest player; a square john, though not necessarily a sucker or pigeon.

Spitballing Cheating method in which a victim is talked into a bad bet because the cheater appears to be betting the same way. The cheater puts up a small amount of money with the victim's large bankroll, then receives a commission from a confederate who wins the bet.

Square john Victim or dupe, especially a naive or very honest-appearing one.

Steer joint Crooked gambling house to which victims are brought by ropers or guided by steerers, who receive a commission or share in the money cheated from the victim.

Submarine Loose-fitting bloomers worn under the clothing to catch chips dropped into the shirt or inside the waistband of trousers (used by dishonest dealers to steal from the house).

Sure-thing man Cheater who takes bets only on events which have been predetermined, so there is no chance to lose.

Where's Buster Brown   Signal to a confederate to switch crooked dice
into the game.

There was, however, one honest form of gambling early in the days of
the Republic—the lottery. In fact, the Revolutionary War itself was a call
for the colonists to help raise $1.5 million by participating in a lottery in
the year 1777.

The pitch was convincing. Here it is documented in *People of Chance*
by John M. Findlay: "It is not doubted but every real friend of his country
will most cheerfully become an adventurer, and that the sale of tickets will
be very rapid, especially as even the unsuccessful adventurer will have the
pleasing reflection of having contributed a degree to the great and glorious
American cause." The "unsuccessful adventurer" (loser) is a euphemism
worthy of today's ad copy writer.

But lotteries had a notable downside. They were a magnet for dishonest
officials and scam artists of every stripe. The real anti-gambling crusades
were stoked by the corruption of the various state lotteries. Often a state
legislature would turn to a private company to run its lottery. In one
such instance in Pennsylvania, "the lottery agents provided the state with
$27,000 annually, but they also grossed over $800,000 per year themselves
on ticket sales of more than $5 million . . . Tales of other abuse circulated,
too, prompting citizens throughout the nation to join the crusade against
lotteries," Findlay writes.

Millions of counterfeit lottery tickets were sold each year; "agents"
operated on the streets or out of fake lottery offices. "One such agent
during the 1820s was teenager P.T. Barnum, who learned some of his
showmanship from various schemes and also discovered by selling tickets
to foolish buyers that 'such bipeds as "humbugs" certainly existed before
I attained my majority.'"

Between 1830 and 1860 every state in the union banned lotteries.
By 1890 the Federal government had stepped in and made all forms of
gambling illegal. Undaunted, gamblers went underground, some opening

ornate casinos known as "splendid hells." Nevada legalized gambling in 1931. The states got back in the lottery business in 1964, starting with New Hampshire. Although the lotteries are probably not rigged, some states have adopted questionable advertising tactics. The Illinois lottery, for example, posted a billboard in a Chicago slum, reading: "This could be your ticket out." It's no secret that most lottery players are those who can afford it least.

Chapter 6

Moderation

The compulsive gambler wants something like love or quiescence, and in his best moments only gets money. He wants to fill some emptiness, and he pushes his bets so far he ends up with greater emptiness, perhaps an emptiness that has an odd measure of solace in it: he can delude himself that he knows its sources. —Stephen Dunn

INSIDE A BOX OF MEMORABILIA I found a wad of War Time Food and Gasoline Ration stamps and the program from the 1941 Kentucky Derby. "A bunch of us guys drove all night to Louisville," my father recalls. His handicapping skills were dubious even then. (His forte, as noted, was dice.) Passing up the eventual winner, Whirlaway, my father bet an also-ran called Robert Morris. Whirlaway went on to capture the Preakness and Belmont Stakes for the Triple Crown.

I was born the next year. Shortly after that, the family moved to Los Angeles. "I had $13 in my pocket," my father says. "I didn't know what I was going to do. I had passed my physical. The war was on. Then Roosevelt announced that fathers over 31 would not be inducted. I had just turned 31. I was mad as hell because I knew there was a lot of gambling in the army."

My father's apartment hunting hit a snag each time: "no kids allowed." But help was on the way. His family loaned my parents $500, and my mother's parents came through with the other $500, for a down payment on a tidy two-bedroom, $5,000 house on South Holt Avenue. When they first approached their new dwelling my five-year-old brother whispered to my mother: "Do they take kids here?"

Just holding onto the new home and watching the appreciation soar would have made my father a rich man in two decades. But that kind of action was much too slow. So he drove a milk truck, then moved up to route man for Eagle Bakery, and found gambling action God knows where. Some Saturdays, he'd pick me up at home at dawn and I'd get to accompany him on his route, sitting high up in the truck cab. A schmoozer without peer, he'd stop repeatedly for coffee and we'd sit at the counter while he chatted with the help and early morning diners. Riding shotgun throughout LA in the whitebread Truman-Eisenhower era was a giddy sensation as I watched my extrovert father charm one and all.

I tended to be somber. Relatives would constantly ask me: why don't you ever smile? I had no ready answer. I was rejected by the school "in crowd." My self-esteem plummeted. Then something happened. As our fifth-grade class was being marched downstairs to the library, the teacher reprimanded us: "Stop!" she said sternly. "You children sound like a bunch of horses going down these stairs." As soon as she got out of earshot I heard myself bellow: "And there goes the old gray mare." Laughter erupted, echoed through the hallway, reverberated off the walls, buoyed me. I became a wisecracker, mistaking laughter for acceptance.

One memorable day at the Eagle Bakery a worker handed me a fresh glazed donut, still steaming. It was like biting into a sugary cloud.

Out in the parking lot, the taste turned sour when my father ordered me, "Stand over there." I obeyed, shooting a glance at him and the other drivers, now on their knees in a small circle. Gee, I thought, they're awfully big for playing marbles.

Of course, these marbles were square and had little dots on them. One of their crap games was later busted up by undercover cops; it was my father's first of several gambling related arrests.

* * *

Once I told a girl in sixth grade that I was going home for lunch and then heading off to Las Vegas. She noticed my fingers crossed behind my back. "You're making that up," she said. The truth was, I'd had my fingers crossed all day to insure that the trip plans didn't fall apart. They didn't.

I still remember my first walk through a Las Vegas casino. I'm enchanted by the clanging slot machines, the lush maroon carpets, the shiny silver dollars and the gamblers' exuberance as they play dice. A pit boss jokes to me, "Get your bet down!" I'm eight years old, my head spinning with delight. Suddenly a slot machine explodes in bells and rains silver dollars into a bucket and onto the floor; the player, a huge woman with platinum hair, leaps up and down, elated, grabbing the silver. I stop wide-eyed and stare. My father takes in my fascination. "Anything is OK," he whispers, "in moderation." I miss the point—and, of course, the irony.

Vegas then was like the Land of Oz, compared to the dull gray Kansas of Los Angeles. We'd sit ringside at dinner shows, dazzled by Sinatra, Sammy Davis Jr, Judy Garland, the Mills Brothers and lesser stars like Peter Lind Hayes and Mary Healey. Once, as Judy Garland was belting "The Trolley Song," a leggy cigarette girl approached our table and bent down, revealing rolling cleavage. My father and I absorbed the sensual treat, then locked eyes, a silent message passing from father to son. I tingled with anticipation for s-e-x.

I would visit Vegas as a child and later as a teenager with false ID, a young adult, with girl friends, wives, and ultimately family reunions. But Vegas in 1950, when I started going there with my father, was still primitive, including the Last Frontier, which featured bumper cars and other carnival-style diversions for kids. My brother and I rode them, unaware that we were present at the creation of a financial boom that would last into the next century.

It was an amazing cast of characters that oversaw Vegas growth from desert dust to a twenty-first century phantasmagoria. Meyer Lansky and Bugsy Siegel lit the torch in 1946 with the first ornate palace in the desert, the Flamingo Hotel.

"What I had in mind," the prescient Lansky would later say, "was to build the greatest, most luxurious hotel casino in the world and invite people from all over America—maybe the high rollers from all over the world—to come and spend their money there." Siegel's fate was sealed when he overspent the Flamingo's budget by several million. The handsome mobster was gunned down in Beverly Hills before the year was out. But months later the Flamingo flourished, as did the other Strip hotels built in the 50s—Desert Inn, Sands, Showboat, New Frontier, Royal Nevada, Dunes and the luxurious Tropicana. Las Vegas was drawing 8 million visitors a year, who managed to lose a reported $200 million.

There were no illusions in Las Vegas about who owned the hotels and had profit skimming down to an art. The mobsters employed "fronts" as owners. But a spate of gangland warfare in the 1950s threatened the enterprise. Racketeer Frank Costello was shot and wounded in 1957; the next year Riviera owner Gus Greenbaum had his throat cut. His wife suffered the same brutal death. Nevada responded with a commission to regulate gambling, keeping undesirables from getting licenses. This was only mildly successful, since the mobsters owned politicians and gaming officials alike.

Las Vegas was poised for phenomenal growth, but finding large investors was not easy. The ubiquitous Moe Dalitz, the mobster who hailed from Cleveland and owned the Desert Inn, stepped in and arranged a meeting between local banker Thomas Parry and Teamster President James Hoffa, whose pension fund was tapped for $200 million to funnel into Las Vegas hotel expansion. The city prospered.

By the mid-sixties Las Vegas was ready for its next incarnation. The reclusive billionaire Howard Hughes snuck into town and holed up on the ninth floor of the Desert Inn. When Dalitz tried to evict him to make room for the high rollers, Hughes bought the hotel. That merely whetted the billionaire's appetite. "How many more of these toys are available?" Hughes asked his point man Robert Maheu, according to Denton and Morris in *The Money and the Power*. "We need a few more." Hughes quickly acquired the Sands, Frontier, Landmark and Silver Slipper. Four years later, Hughes, now a ghostly apparition addicted to painkillers and exhibiting bizarre behavior, left town. Las Vegas had passed the Corporate Gambling Act, giving the town a sense of legitimacy that would hasten such big money players as Kirk Kerkorian and Steve Wynn, who would battle for supremacy. Meanwhile, Vegas corporations would invest billions in theme hotel mania, creating the Luxor, Paris, Venice, Rio, San Remo, and New York New York, so "authentic" that steam rises from the manholes.

Most Vegas visitors are willingly seduced. The question seldom asked is how many compulsive and problem gamblers are needed to keep Bellagio's massive desert lake shimmering, the lava of Caesars Palace flowing, and millions of neon bulbs glowing? Casino officials maintain that they "don't target compulsives. They target repeat customers." Adds the president of the American Gaming Association in *Bad Bet* by Timothy O'Brien: "This is a very competitive business. People can't continue to gamble if they are compulsives. They eventually lose all of their money."

Notes author O'Brien: "Compulsives, of course, have found myriad ways, including theft, to raise gambling funds once their cash runs out. And there is good reason to believe that compulsive and problem gambling is a bigger revenue source than the industry cares to acknowledge."

"My concern is that this is not a minor issue on the revenue side," says William Eadington, an economics professor at the University of Nevada at Reno and a leading authority on gambling. "I think if you restrain people who are compulsives or problem gamblers it would have a very significant impact on the revenue of casinos."

Once you pull up the rug on "the gambling issue," you're awash in claims, counterclaims and research results that prove Mark Twain's dictum, "There are three levels of falsehoods: lies, damned lies, and statistics." Translation: whoever funds the study is likely to get the results sought. As noted earlier, Congress took up the issue with its National Gambling Impact Study Commission. The *Los Angeles Times* reported an intriguing fact left out of the report. "The commission administered a preliminary survey outside two Las Vegas casinos. The result suggested that 30 percent of the casinos' clientele showed indications of being problem gamblers." Outraged gambling industry officials found fault with the survey's methodology and got it supressed.

In my own random, nonscientific survey, conducted in 2002 aboard a public bus on The Strip, I noticed that a significant number of couples were arguing bitterly over money lost. The husbands frequently turned silent, unable to explain how they vastly exceeded their loss limits.

As we grew up, my brother developed the gambling bug too, but he remained rational. He never lost more than he could afford. When he was busted, he quit. My father, however, saw a losing session as a sign to ratchet up his bets, and later, so did I. It was the clearest sign of the addict, known as "chasing." The gambler pumps more and more money in a futile attempt to get even. Later on, the addict begins to harbor the illusion that when he hits that big win—recouping all his losses—he will stop gambling. He clings to the fallacy that gambling is about winning. It's not. It's the adrenaline rush of playing that keeps you on the treadmill.

Part 2

GAMBLING DEMONS

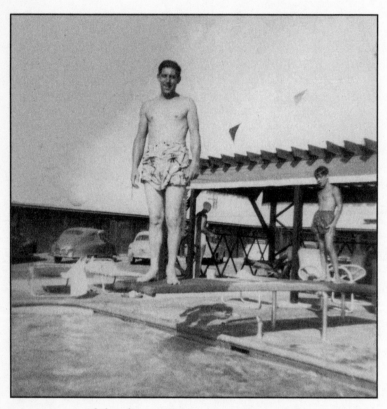

Phil and Burt Dragin in Las Vegas, 1950

Chapter 7

First Pilgrimage

When I think of this artificial vividness plunked down in the midst of the most primitive part of the world, I have a curious sense of Las Vegas's history—the covered wagons so little a while ago, and now it's all air-conditioned and neon. I find a wonderful excess underfoot. Everything, you see, is arranged here. And yet, I suspect, there's a tragic side.

—Noel Coward

ON OUR FIRST VEGAS FAMILY PILGRIMAGE IN 1950, we were ensconced at the Rancho Anita, a nondescript motel off The Strip. Somewhere in my parents' shoe box of black-and-white snapshots is one of the Rancho Anita with an inked arrow pointing to "our car." We made our way to the newly minted Flamingo Hotel. The exterior was a riot of neon; the garish facade had pink bubbles rising toward the desert sky. The scorching heat was dry and unforgiving. But inside the Flamingo it was air conditioned! The contrast worked its magic. Unbeknownst to me, a habit had taken root.

Years later, when my father realized I was following in his risky footsteps, he shared the casinos' best kept secret: craps offers the only correct odds bet. Hence my father's paternal wisdom was summed up in six words: "Always back up your line bets." A line bet is a wager on the "pass line" for which the player is paid at even money; on the first roll of the dice the bet can be ended in one of five ways. A seven or eleven is a winner; two, three or twelve is a loser. The remaining numbers—four, five, six, eight, nine and ten—are "points." Assuming the shooter has not thrown a natural (7

43

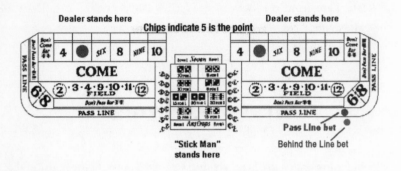

Dealer stands here

Chips indicate 5 is the point

or 11) or crapped out (2, 3 or 12), he continues throwing the dice trying to make his point. From here on the bet is settled in only one of two ways; the player makes the point and wins, or throws a seven and loses. When the shooter (or anyone at the crap table) gets a point he can put money "behind the pass line" and get paid the correct odds, depending on his point. If the point is four or ten, he gets paid 2 to 1 for the behind the line bet; if the point is five or nine, he gets paid 3 to 2; and if the point is six or eight, he gets paid at 6 to 5. These are the only bets paid at true odds in the casino. The dice table dealers seldom tout these bets, but do talk up others where the house has a decided advantage.

A math whiz named Jess Marcum in 1980 figured out just how vital it is for a crap shooter to "hit and run." Marcum concluded that "a craps player who wagered just $1 every bet for two months would have only one chance in 2 trillion to win $1,000 before he lost $1,000. On the other hand, by decreasing his exposure at the craps table to just 25 minutes and wagering $200 every bet, that same gambler would improve his odds to 1.15 to 1." Marcum has presented the most potent possible example of the casinos' "grind 'em out" theory. Make larger and fewer bets and, he shows, the odds against you (in the case of craps) are barely greater than even money.

Accordingly, as a casino guest, you are clearly welcome for as long as you want to stay. If you're a slot player, you're even more welcome; slots have become the biggest profit makers for the casinos. The very decor of the casino, including the mirrors, is designed to disorient the slot players and keep them from wandering off. Writes Gary Rivlin in the *New York Times Magazine:* "Nearly 40 million Americans played a slot machine in 2003, according to an annual survey of casino gambling conducted by Harrah's Entertainment. Every day in the United States, slot machines take in, on average, more than $1 billion in wagers. Most of that money will be paid back to players, but so great is the hold from slot machines that collectively the games gross more annually than McDonalds, Wendys, Burger King and Starbucks combined. All told, North American casinos took in $30 billion from slots in 2003—an amount that dwarfs the $9 billion in tickets sold in North American movie theaters that year."

In his book *The Luck Business,* former *Boston Globe* columnist Robert Goodman observes that gambling "is where some Ph.D.s write about treating neuropsychological disorders of addicted gamblers, while others research behavior modification techniques that will encourage more people to gamble. It is backed by sophisticated state-of-the-art marketing and ever-fresh enticements—where mathematicians develop new games, 'theming' consultants create mythical dream worlds, and demographic experts conduct segmentation surveys to target the socioeconomic profiles of potential players."

My father the truck driver metamorphosed into his private fantasy in Vegas. Still trim, hair slicked down, dapper, he would stride up to the dice table, coolly acknowledge the pit boss' greeting, then drop a hundred dollar bill onto the green felt and announce "ten plays." He had become George Raft!

We did manage one non-Vegas vacation, a train trip to Cleveland. Dad remained home. I was ten, my brother Bill 14 and already an accomplished gin rummy player. We were seated in the lounge car when two older boys asked if we were interested in "a little gambling action." My brother assented with feigned deliberation. I ordered some fruit juice concoction that looked alcoholic.

When my mother walked into the lounge car and saw her ten-year-old playing cards and "drinking," she came unglued. She would tell the story for years. "There was Burt, playing cards and drinking!" Bill and I managed to beat the hustlers out of almost five dollars. "They thought they were going to take us," my brother proclaimed. For me, it was the highlight of brotherhood.

As the older sibling, Bill was aware of the family dysfunction. Once, after a bitter parental battle over Topic A (Dad's gambling losses), there ensued a lengthy silence. Bill made a potent pronouncement: "I don't see why you got married in the first place." More silence.

Later on I'd wonder about Mom—devoted to her kids, yet her role with her husband was more complex: enabler, antagonist, co-dependent. And Dad? It occurred to me that his problem might be the same as Hickey's, the wayward protagonist in Eugene O'Neil's *The Iceman Cometh,* whose wife, Hickey announced with seething dismay, "always forgave me." My parents appeared to be doing some weird dance, as if they were sentenced to marriage and had to endure hard time. Had they been in the "old country," I can imagine an arranged marriage in which my father viewed his bride's dowry as his gambling stake.

Blossoming out of his teens—with frequent trips to Vegas, Santa Anita and other gambling venues—my brother saw his love of gambling surpassed by his love of food. "The worst four words in the English language," he revealed to me at a sumptuous Vegas hotel buffet line, are, "All You Can Eat." He couldn't resist the calories, but could the gambling. He became an accountant and raised a family.

Bill was too practical to be a compulsive gambler. He purchased single shares of stock in Santa Anita racetrack for each family member because each included passes for the exclusive clubhouse. To this day I receive my quarterly dividend check for about 20 cents and the annual statement with four clubhouse passes, which I dutifully mail off to Bill. Asked recently about his decades of recreational gambling, Bill replied: "My big regret is all that time wasted."

Chapter 8

High School Highlight

If you win, and you're not excited, then you haven't won at all.
—Jack Gollehon

HIGH SCHOOL, FOR ME, WAS SOCIAL ANGST AND QUICK EXITS. During my senior year I was on "four/four," half a day at school, half a day allegedly working at my father's hamburger stand. I made the acquaintance of gamblers. They were not hard to find. My most memorable day at LA's Alexander Hamilton High School was neither the senior prom nor homecoming (both of which I missed) but an off-campus escapade at Hollywood Park racetrack. Trapped in Mrs. Plummer's American history class, I perused the *Daily Racing Form.* Plummer might wax eloquent on Washington, Jefferson, Adams, and Lincoln, but I was versed in Arcaro, Longdon, Neves, Valenzuela, and Shoemaker—the diminutive athletes who guided the 1,200-pound thoroughbreds around the track. The classroom was static. The clock was still, then lurched forward on the minute. The teacher had placed a sign under it: "Time Passes. Will You?"

While Plummer praised the patriot Tom Paine, a bay colt called Danny James leaped off the page of my racing form. A hall pass got me as far as the school perimeter. I shot a glance at the lunch area; the cliques were already holding court. The colorful club jackets documented the social caste system. I longed to be a Knight but an invitation to pledge never came. The untouchables ate alone, feigning lack of interest. I squeezed through the broken gate. My '51 sky-blue Ford roared to life. Twenty minutes later I turned onto Arbor Vitae, the gorgeously named street that took you through the seamy end of Inglewood and into the massive racetrack parking lot.

A burly cop spotted me approaching a stranger near the racetrack entrance. I was looking for someone to play my "father" so I could get in. I found a candidate, but seconds later the cop was in the guy's face saying, "You know you're contributing to the delinquency of a minor?" The guy shrugged and walked in alone.

The cop lowered his bulk and put his oily face near mine: "You are not getting in here today." Was there a more enticing invitation to a game of cat and mouse? I stowed my red sweater in the car, stayed alert and slipped in through a different gate.

Once inside the racetrack grounds, I felt the electric thrill as I spotted the green tote board, heard the brass-buttoned bugler ushering the horses onto the track, and wandered among the sun-drenched hopeful. Some were boozing, some were chiding young ones, but all clung to their colorful racetrack programs. Ecstatic children were scooping up handfuls of discarded parimutuel tickets, later to be checked against the results in hopes of finding a winner. (Why aren't these kids in school, I wondered, oblivious to the irony of my thought.)

Meanwhile, in the track's infield, the white-gowned goose girl strolled among the colorful fauna. What a scene! Strangers who would ignore each other on the street talked hunches like best friends. Then came the booming staccato voice of announcer Harry Hensen: "The horses are coming onto the track for the fifth race at six furlongs." My pulse quickened.

Near the betting windows, I caught the rank odor of racetrack hot dogs, beer, and thick cigarette smoke. People were scurrying about: the old, the young, the desperate, the touts, and the women who seemed oblivious to their crying children. As the race time drew near, this cramped space turned even more frantic. In fact, this scene was a recurring dream. I'm in the betting line with a sure thing but time runs out. The race starts and that hideous bell rings.

The bell itself was once the angle of an imaginative racetrack hustler. Since it rang just after the horses broke from the gate, he figured he'd have a split second to see which horse grabbed the lead. If that horse was a front runner—a frequent winner with a good break—he'd place the bet just before the bell rang. This entailed posting several cronies from the betting window to someone with a view of the track to give the signal. Apparently they had some success, because the track changed the policy: no action after the gate opens.

I keep an eye out for Mitch, my horseplayer guru who at age 16 had been stopped by the cops at the payoff windows with $900 in winning tickets. Mitch was a social misfit with an all-consuming love for horse-race gambling and a phenomenal ability to win. An accountant by day, Mitch was an uncanny handicapper. He thought of little else but the horses. He was bulky, had lousy teeth and seldom cut his unruly brown hair. He drove a battered Chevy, wore the same faded Levi's and black T-shirt day after day. Tucked under his arm—always—was the *Daily Racing Form*.

Mitch had no inhibitions. One day he's sitting in the grandstand when a friend, several rows away, asks how he's doing. "Still a virgin," Mitch yells, indicating he has yet to cash a ticket. When anyone sought his opinion on a horse he thought had no chance, Mitch had a two-word summary: "Dog meat." Mitch was now around 20 and already a legend. He would later own racehorses, become a successful CPA and grow wild salt-and-pepper hair and beard. Social convention would never dent his philosophy of life: play the angle (an "edge" over other players).

Once at Santa Anita I witnessed Mitch's betting savvy. We had just parked and were heading for the entrance gate.

"This is interesting," Mitch said, scanning the parking lot.

"What?"

Mitch had noticed a slew of cars with Arizona plates. He checked the *Daily Racing Form* and noticed a filly in the first race, a Phoenix import. Since the race was for maidens—horses who've never won—Mitch suspected the Arizona crowd had more than a casual interest in the first race. Mitch played his hunch. The Phoenix filly won by six lengths.

Like an underage tout, I loiter near the $5 window. The first person to make eye contact gets my request: "Can you bet number seven for me?" A matronly type takes the fiver and checks the board. "Twenty-five to one," she mumbles handing me the win ticket. This is no place for a teenager to get caught placing a bet.

From low in the grandstand I watch through binoculars as the horses are led into the starting gate, the jockeys' bright racing silks—pink, green, orange, black—flapping in the spring breeze. For an instant the crowd noise ceases; all listen for Hensen's authoritative voice: "The-flag-is-up." Pause. "Annnnnnd there they go!" The gate cracks open and the horses are suspended in air, soon to fulfill their destiny—and ours.

They charge forward with legs a tangled blur, making a faraway thunderous sound, kicking up mounds of loose dirt. Danny James breaks well and the jockey quickly hustles him to the inside to save ground. From up here they look like dominoes magically pushed along the track. But from down near the rail, where I often stand, you see the horses' raw power—sinewy muscles glistening—and stunning speed as they skim the brown turf, the jockeys' delicate hands restraining these massive animals until the moment comes to unleash them.

The horses start out way beyond the infield, far from the spectators. Danny James, in flashing green silks, is running just off the pace, about fifth, in a good spot. He is a strong closer but was blocked behind horses in his last two starts. I'm hopeful because he's still up with the leaders.

As the horses go into the turn for the home stretch, the crowd responds with its inevitable roar. That's merely the start of a crescendo.

When I see Danny James starting his move on the outside, my binoculars locked on him, I experience the supreme gambler's thrill. The jockey cracks the whip once and Danny James responds with a fluid burst of speed. "Turning for home," Hensen intones, "it's Danny James gaining ground on the outside . . ." Nothing else Hensen says is audible once the horses are in front of the stands—the stretch drive. The cheering crowd overwhelms everything.

Danny James appears to pass the number three horse, the favorite, and take the lead, but the favorite isn't through yet. Both jockeys go to the whip, squeezing more life from their mounts. The two horses battle, stride for stride, nose and nose, all the way to the finish wire. I'm hoarse from yelling, my stomach in knots. The two horses streak under the wire, the jockeys now upright as they await the outcome, which surprises no one. Says Hensen: "The result is a photo finish." My heart throbs through the five-minute delay, my mind awash in unbidden images . . . Mrs. Plummer and Tom Paine, the Knights' cool black and silver jackets, Sally Bayers' lush blonde hair, the dent I put in my father's Oldsmobile.

Then: "The result is official. The winner is number seven, Danny James . . ." I'm leaping, screaming, squeezing the winning ticket. I'm alive! For my $5 I get $130 . . . but more importantly I get a spectacular stretch drive I can replay in my mind forever. It never occurs to me there is a downside to such elation. But there is. Decades later I discover that my brain still hungers for the Danny James high—again and again.

Chapter 9

My Father's Decade

Winning and losing and the expectations therefrom are diverting. I conceive there would be no pleasure properly so called if a man were sure to win. It is the reconciling of uncertainty to our desires that creates the satisfaction. —Frederick Brandt

THE SIXTIES MAY HAVE BEEN TURBULENT FOR THE NATION, but for my father, the decade started off in sublime fashion. He bought a new metallic silver T-bird; he joined the Beverly Hills Health Club (the best $600 wager of his life). He purchased his clothes at Tavelmen's in Beverly Hills. He took his family to eateries on La Cienega's pricey Restaurant Row. Once at Lawry's Prime Rib restaurant (not one hundred yards from Dolores Drive-Inn, where my father had until recently delivered bread at 5 a.m.), I heard my father kibitzing with a health club crony as we waited for our table. "Boy, you've got to have a good front in this town," my father said. I'm thinking: What are you, a movie producer? You own a hamburger stand in Culver City. Later on it would occur to me that a "good front" was necessary when you put the "touch" on someone.

My father visited Cleveland with his pride intact, a "business mogul" after his inauspicious start at Amato's Pool Hall and its clientele destined for prison or early death. He charmed the relatives, flashing photos of his hamburger stand not two blocks from MGM Studios—a locale that provided a whiff of glamour. Some minor celebrities did make it over to Phil's Drive Inn, including songwriter Johnny Mercer and the kid who played Rusty on *Make Room for Daddy,* the Danny Thomas sitcom. Then out of nowhere one day Elvis Presley, the King himself, came driving up in an Isetta, a tiny three-wheel vehicle. A crowd materialized. My mother waited on Elvis, who ordered several hamburgers to go. And not only did my mother not receive one of the gifts Elvis was reputed to bestow on strangers—she mistakenly undercharged him!

So there was my father in his late 40s: handsome and lean still, a snappy dresser who charmed the waitresses, always tipped well, identified with the working stiff, and felt sorry for the "average guy on the street." In a sense, my father and I led parallel lives. We performed society's minimal demands—junior college classes in my case, running a hamburger stand in his—but our thoughts were always locked on the next bet. That was the only way to stir the juices. For me, it became Gardena, an enclave of poker clubs about thirty minutes out the San Diego Freeway. I dated frequently, but halfway through the movie or party or dinner I'd take furtive glances at my watch, wondering how many more minutes before I'd be at the poker tables, watching the cards slide across the green felt into my eager hands.

I favored the Normandie Club, playing $5 limit lowball draw. A startling range of characters showed up, eagerly paying the $1 "collection" every thirty minutes. That was before poker clubs employed dealers. One slightly inebriated guy proclaimed—in mid-deal—that "Jesus Christ is my brother-in-law." After spilling the cards on the floor he explained that his sister was a nun.

There were few fights, although floormen in loud sport jackets were there to adjudicate any dispute. The clubs employed "props," or proposition players, who were paid to fill in when a game was short of players. The money they won or lost was their own. We knew who they were and respected their play. I even toyed with becoming a prop player some day. But the boredom on their faces steered me clear of such ambition.

Mostly it was the same faces, playing the same level games (starting at

fifty cents/one dollar) night after night. Dawn brought massive depression
for the losers. The clubs closed at 5 a.m. Frequently I found myself broke,
disgusted, exhausted, staring at the sunrise through bloodshot eyes.

I was oblivious to how many of the players were addicts, bedding
down in local flophouses, abusing alcohol and any other means of escape.
Almost four decades later would I learn through a *Los Angeles Times* article
on compulsive gambling just how lethal these Gardena clubs could be.

The newspaper profiled a Gardena habitue named Rex, "who shares
floor space in cheap motels with other compulsive gamblers, comforting
himself with delusional dreams of jackpots that will magically wipe away
three decades of wreckage." Rex lost "his marriage, his home, his Cadillac,
his clothes, his diamond ring. Not least of all, in the card clubs of Southern
California, he has lost his pride." The most staggering fact about Rex was his
former life: "Articulate, intellectual, he talks about existential philosophy, the
writings of Camus and Sartre. He was once an editor at Random House."

The first semester at Los Angeles City College was a shock. Professors
expected work. I dropped out and joined an army reserve ordnance company. Somehow I made it to the golf course most days. Inside the barracks
were dice and poker. Some sharpies shot dice on a blanket, even finding
a few takers. I knew enough to avoid a game where the dice "roll" rather
than "spin," giving the shooter a large measure of control. The stud poker
games were embarrassing. Some neophytes bet stiff hands—hands that
had no chance of winning, as was obvious by their face-up cards. More
experienced guys took advantage of them. I wasn't that hard up for cash.

And then there was Douglas, the most taciturn, self-contained private
in the barracks—until he picked up the dice. Pumped to life by two num-
bered cubes, he'd let loose with every dice cliché known to man—"Little
Joe," "Up Jumped the Devil," "Niner from Carolina," "Snake Eyes"—and
he could be heard through the barracks and probably on the other side of
the post. When the game ended, he deflated like a popped balloon, return-
ing to his introverted self.

Halfway through the Sixties, my father's empire began to crumble. He had built a second hamburger stand at 47th and Figueroa, not far from notorious South-Central LA—but also near Inglewood and Hollywood Park. Perhaps my father should have taken it as an omen at his Culver City hamburger stand when a guy came to the window and asked if he could place a bet on a horse. Incredibly, my father agreed. The guy came to the back door and asked my father if he had the day's sports page. My father obliged, the guy circled the horse, and my father said "Okay."

"You're under arrest," the undercover cop said. My father tried to explain that he was going to place the bet at the track—which might have been true. But the cop ignored the plea and made the pinch. My father paid a fine and later learned through the grapevine that this cop had a rep as pure slimeball.

Hollywood Park was gobbling up my father's profits, and soon he turned to loan sharks to keep him afloat. He had plummeted to the "one big score" theory that would allow him to wipe out his debts. Predictably, it never happened. We sold the house and moved to an apartment in Culver City. It was a stunning revelation. Gambling brought not only bitter parental arguments but a financial reversal that took our family's household and its memories. "No pets in the apartment," I'm told. Crushed, I'm forced to part with Queenie, a sweet shepard-collie mix who was my best friend.

Soon hamburger stand number one, then number two were sucked away. Said my father decades later: "Watts went down the drain and I went down the drain with it."

I was not privy to the financial squeeze my father endured. My parents split up, and the next thing I knew my father was driving a Helm's Bakery truck in an area not far from my grade school. (As a typical self-absorbed teenager, I thought little of the impact of their separation and the loneliness it must have caused them both.) Another yellow truck, this one for hawking bread, donuts, and pies to the homes along the way. It was a job for immigrants and the uneducated. My father was robbed at gunpoint for the pittance he carried. But what really galled him on this job were the teenagers who ridiculed him. I almost wish my father could have morphed into his teenage self with his gangster persona. The local toughs would have run like hell.

My father's downward spiral continued—menial jobs, dead-end jobs, no jobs. The worst was running a greasy spoon in downtown LA. I paid a visit to this nightmare scene, which could have been the locale in the film *L.A. Confidential* where the detectives wander in to discover carnage among the grime. This was the first time I felt genuine fear for my father's life. Any minute I expected a drug-addled creep with a gun to stagger in and demand all the cash, ready to put a bullet through anyone who flinched. Did my father carry a gun? I didn't want to know.

So my father's working these jobs, trying to get back with my mother, and meanwhile we're both still gambling. My father has friends, many of whom hang out at a bowling alley, another of my father's passions. I'm moving obliquely toward a degree in English, working a flunky job for the Los Angeles County Counsel, living in a $75 a month decrepit one-room apartment in Palms, a bedroom community just off the Santa Monica Freeway.

The tuition-free junior college classes were a popular justification for such a lifestyle. I'd run into friends with a similar gig. "What are you majoring in?" Econ, or Poli Sci or, in my case, English. No one pressed further for your plans. You were in college; that was enough. We'd spot one another frequently at the racetrack or Gardena. Of course, I had friends at UCLA and one in Berkeley who had real plans.

But I did get stoked twice in a junior college philosophy class. First there was Blaise Pascal (1623-62), credited with mapping out the first theory of probability. My gambling research would reveal that Pascal was beaten a century earlier by a physician/scholar/compulsive gambler named Gerolamo Cordano. Pascal's renown was without question. But I was most intrigued by his famous "Wager," wherein he argues that betting on the existence of God is the only choice for the believer and the nonbeliever alike. Pascal's reasoning goes like this:

- If one bets on God and believes, then there are two possible outcomes:
  - (1) God exists: one enjoys an eternity of bliss. Or
  - (2) God does not exist: one loses very little.

- On the other hand if one bets against God and wins, one gains very little. But if one loses that bet, the consequences may be horrendous.

In my view, Pascal has simply offered a brief for the percentage play. Scholars, of course, read profound philosophical meaning into Pascal's Wager. Writes Jeff Jordan in *Gambling on God: Essays on Pascal's Wager,* "A Pascalian wager is a decision situation in which the possible gain or benefit involved in one of the outcomes swamps all the others." For the compulsive gambler, I hesitate to point out, the only wager that swamps all others is not wagering at all.

But it was Zeno's paradox that intrigued me most. Zeno of Elea (490-430 BC) argued the most outrageous positions through *reductio ad absurdum.* For example, Zeno posited that a runner could never finish a race. Why? Because he gets halfway down the course and continues running only to complete half the distance remaining and then the next half and on into infinity.

I would have loved to have been sitting at the Santa Anita finish wire with Zeno when my favorite racehorse, Silky Sullivan, was in his prime. Silky was odd; he seemed to wait in the starting gate until all the horses blasted out, then he would casually join the race. But Silky had incredible stamina and a sixth sense about the location of the finish line, because he would pass the entire field and just barely win the race. This, I'm sure, would have cost Zeno some big dough, were he a philosopher willing to back up his paradox theory with cash. Such were the idle thoughts that occupied me during my first run at college. A few years later I'd return, having mastered Academic Survival—the unwritten rules of getting by.

But mostly I—like my father—was absorbed by the fast moving betting seasons—baseball, football, basketball and horses almost year round. And, of course, the casinos with their booze and glitz and 24-hour action.

The one time I felt genuine dismay toward my father over gambling happened during the mid-Sixties and involved a football wager, an instance of my catching an "in-between." The bookies often had wildly different point spreads, and the smart bettor would shop around. I knew my father had bet the underdog football team and gotten 13 points. The bookie I bet with had made the other team a nine-point favorite. This was a huge difference.

To catch an in-between you bet the underdog and take the points and bet the favorite and give the points. If the score falls in the middle of the spreads—in between—you win both bets. If it doesn't you win one and lose one, costing you additionally ten percent of the losing bet, the bookie's interest (or "vig"). I met my father at the bowling alley and asked him to bet $200 for me on the underdog. I'll never forget his enigmatic reply: "I've got my own problems." No bet. Of course, the score fell in the middle and I blew an easy $400!

Somewhere in my consciousness was a blurred vision of the future— maybe I'd wind up a derelict at Gardena, or some drifter slinking from racetrack to racetrack. I knew of such pathetic characters. And I had watched James Caan in *The Gambler,* writer James Toback's paean to the gambling addict as college English professor, intellectual yet unable to stop his precipitous descent into hell. Says Axel, the film's protagonist, about gambling: "It's just something I like to do. I like the uncertainty of it. I like the threat of losing, the idea that I could lose but somehow I won't because I don't want to. And I love winning even though it never lasts . . . If all my bets were safe there just wouldn't be any juice."

Nineteen sixty-eight was a pivotal year. I was in college for real, actually pursuing a bachelor's degree in English, yet unemployed. I perused the want ads. My mother was sending me care packages, my father calling with job tips. And there, in the middle of the *Los Angeles Times* classifieds, was a sentence in tiny type that would change my life: "Wanted. Editorial trainee for newspaper chain."

The job paid only $75 a week, yet the waiting room was packed with eager candidates. I filled out the forms and awaited a call back. An entré to the newspaper world! I wanted it desperately. My mother gave me sound though distasteful advice: "Go back there," she said. "Pester them. Let them know you want the job." I did so. "Okay," said Tony Scott, the editor. "We'll give you a two-week trial." It was like hitting an inside straight. The job included covering lunchtime speakers at the now infamous Ambassador Hotel on Wilshire Boulevard and even led to writing a theater review column.

I parlayed the newspaper job into a future by acquiring society's vaunted tickets—a bachelor's in English and then, while still working, a masters in journalism at USC. The thrusts of gambling losses weren't so painful. I could rationalize that I was on my way toward "a career."

I met Sandy through Howard, a mutual friend. She lived in San Francisco, and we soon began spending the weekends together, alternating jetting to the other. Sandy belonged to a ski group that booked a spectacular cabin for the season at Lake Tahoe. A ten-minute drive took you across the majestic Nevada state line to South Shore and a passel of neon monster hotel/casinos—Harrah's, Harvey's, Caesar's, High Sierra. They never closed, blasting air conditioning in the summer, heat in the winter. The free drinks were always cold.

The ski group members preferred socializing in the lodge; I had other priorities. "It's too bad you can't ski right to the casinos," someone cracked. Sandy joined me at least once at a casino, and her comment is etched in my brain: "You've already gambled ten dollars," she said. "Why do you need to gamble more?" She stumped me. (Because I'm addicted?) I made a mental note to share her observation with my father. He loved it. Both of us knew blowing ten bucks was practically a win.

Old joke: "How did you do at the track?"

"I broke even. And boy did I need it."

* * *

Sandy and I got married—but not for long. Gambling was not the issue. Things just . . . fell apart. But now I was living in the Bay Area. (My selective memory was tested 34 years later when Sandy and I met for dinner. She recalled a casino dispute—she wanted us to leave—in which I raved about gambling: "This is the only thing in life that gives me any joy.")

My search for a reporting or teaching position in the Bay Area landed me at Laney College in Oakland. The teaching job soon went from half-time to full-time. Ready cash! Modest rent! The casinos at Tahoe and Reno, Golden Gate Field racetrack and the card clubs in Emeryville beckoned. Once or twice at Golden Gate Fields was enough. It was a sad spectacle. This was not like the race tracks I was used to, Hollywood Park or Santa Anita, premiere venues where the top-ranked thoroughbreds were treated like royalty. The smaller racetracks, like Golden Gate Fields, often drew unscrupulous owners who bought horses past their prime and filled them full of "bute" (butazolidin), an anti-inflamatory drug that permitted them to run despite severe injuries. Most bettors were oblivious; I wasn't.

Chapter 10

Back from Purgatory

The gambling known as business looks with austere disfavor on the business known as gambling. —Ambrose Bierce

MEANWHILE, MY FATHER HAD STAGGERED BACK FROM PURGATORY. He ended a three-year separation with my mother, having convinced her that his gambling was "under control." But more intriguing was his swift move from unemployment to the job he had been groomed for since the day he stepped off the boat at Ellis Island. His $600 lifetime membership at the Beverly Hills Health Club was about to pay off—big time.

Harry, a friend, tells my father: "I got you a job. Pete wants to see you."

Pete Maroni (a pseudonym) is a Beverly Hills bookie right out of central casting. He's a jet-setter, sharp dresser and smooth talker. Pete spends most days at the Health Club, kibitzing and taking his meals.

My father tells Harry, "I don't know nothing about the booking business. Suppose a guy wants a double parlay or something?" [The parlay is a bet on horses in two or more races—all must win. The winnings from the first horse are bet on the second, the second to the third, and so on. The math can get tricky, which is why bookies keep "parlay books" that include all computations.]

Harry is insistent. "Just talk with him."

Pete and my father have breakfast at the club.

"Pete hadn't started yet," my father says. "He didn't know nothing about horses. I thought he knew what he was talking about."

Pete tells my father: "I want you to start today."

"Start what?"

"Taking bets. It's all numbers."

Pete and my father drive to a dingy apartment complex off Santa Monica Boulevard. My father carries a suitcase to make it look like he's moving in. "The apartment did not look too clean or smell good," my father recalls. "There was a cot. A kitchen. A tiny bathroom. Pete dials a number, tells the caller 'Here he is,' and hands me the phone. Guy says he'll call me back and give me the late scratches. Pete and I go out and buy a scratch sheet." (A scratch sheet is a listing of all the horses running that day with the early scratches.)

The guy on phone is the Back Man. "You're not supposed to know who he is," my father says. The Back Man goes over the late scratches. Then he calls back just before each race and my father gives him the bets, each bettor identified with a code. "First day I got nine or ten calls," my father says. "And I'd give him the bets. After the last race he tells me I can go home."

The second day things did not go as smooth. "Young gal calls and wants to bet number 10 in the third race. I take the bet." The Back Man explodes. "I told you to take the third race off!" (Taking the race "off" means no more bets. The woman had bet a race that had already been run.) "Do you have a red pencil?"

"No."

"*No red pencil!* You're supposed to put a red line through the race so you'll know that it's gone."

My father had used a blue pencil. In truth, he was still worrying about parlays. The Back Man had assumed the woman's bet was a sure thing, she having found a sap who would take a bet after the race had been run. The Back Man phoned the next day.

"He starts to laugh and laugh," my father says. "So I wait until he gets through laughing. Then I say: 'I'd like to know what's so damn funny.'"

"You."

"Me? Why me?"

"I've been in this business thirty years," the Back Man explains, "and no one ever told me the truth before. I always find out later how this guy or that guy had stiffed me. And you told me the truth the first day." (The woman's horse had lost, proving she had not colluded with my father, as the Back Man had suspected.)

Responds my father, "What have I got to lose. I don't expect to be here more than a few days."

Back Man: "Why?"

"I never did it before."

"You didn't tell me that."

"You didn't ask me."

The Back Man softens: "Well, we're going to teach you. You're going to be here for a while."

My father is told to get note pads, several pens and pencils. Finally, my father asks about parlays.

Back Man: "Don't you have a parlay book?"

"No."

"You'll have one tomorrow." The Back Man will be fully visible at the club the next morning where he meets my father for breakfast and gives him a parlay book. He also delves into the finer points of taking bets and working together smoothly.

Pete's timing with his bookmaking venture was flawless. From my father's first day on the job business boomed. "We started adding two or three customers a day," he says. "The Back Man didn't last long. Pete got bigger. Soon I was doing twenty to thirty tickets [bets] a day. The Back Man was getting a percentage. When Pete realizes he's got to give the guy a percentage of everything he figures he doesn't need the guy."

New customers weren't hard to find. Pete would frequent a Beverly

Hills bar, a hangout for the well-heeled. The bartenders would point out potential customers for Pete, for which they would get a finder's fee.

Then in a plot line worthy of Hollywood, one of Pete's customers—an insurance exec who's stuck about $3500—gets shot to death in a bar. The widow doesn't know how she's going to pay. "Don't worry," Pete tells her. Turns out she's a bookkeeper, so Pete makes her the new Back Man. She's on salary, of course. "We back each other up," my father says of the new hire. "Get to be good friends."

After a major squabble with a customer, my father starts tape recording the calls. It's around this time I'm invited to pay him a visit. I park my car and walk apprehensively to the apartment, looking over one shoulder, then the other. The place is mottled stucco with peeling red paint on the steps. I ring the bell and hear my father's voice at its most tentative:

"Who . . . is . . . it?"

"Burt."

Several latches unclick and the door opens slowly. "Come over here," says the man with hair now a distinguished looking gray, white slacks and an electric blue silk shirt worn out to conceal the start of midriff bulge. This is my father, giver of values, such as they are. Yet I can't deny my pride.

There he sits, fulfilling his childhood dream. Pink betting slips spread across his desk like a game of solitaire; a phalanx of yellow pencils, several red pens, a phone and a tape recorder. The only thing missing is a green eyeshade. "Listen," my father says excitedly. He backs up the tape recorder and plays a brief exchange with a major TV star who happens to own racehorses. After the customer makes the bet my father is telling him: "My son is a big fan of yours."

"No kidding. That's great," is the reply. "Tell ya what. Bring him out to the ranch some time." I am duly impressed. My father beams. The visit to the ranch, needless to say, never happens. My father regales me with the finer points of taking bets. "Bartenders get preferential treatment. A guy's drinking, he wants to bet and go. Guy calls from an office, you got time, you can kibitz."

The job also involves payoffs and collections, sans threats. I accompany my father on one of these outings. The first client meets our car at a corner and slips my father an envelope with a wad of hundreds. I glance at my father. Here he is again, in his element—practically glowing—a tiny cog in the billion dollar business of illegal bookmaking. "Right," he says after a quick count. We drive on in anonymity, two certified members of the underworld. By this time he's pulling down $400 a week (tax free, of course) and holiday bonuses of $2,000. Incredibly, my father's own gambling is curtailed. "No time," he says. But there is more to it. Does he get a rush from handling the action, finally having the house advantage? ("Yes," he confessed to me long after retirement. "We were really trying to beat these guys.")

So my father had regained his grip on life—driving to the apartment every day, buying the day's scratch sheet, taking different routes just to keep the cops off his trail. Perhaps in his mind my father was steering that spiffy yellow Stutz Bearcat convertible of his youth. My mother, the stoic enabler, stepped out of her role and became an aggressive money manager, banking the cash. My parents were living rent free in an apartment complex in Pasadena, my mother employed as bookkeeper in the rental office. Bookkeeper and bookmaker, my parents were living a not-quite-kosher version of the American dream.

My LA visits always included father-and-son time at the Club. It was glorious to see him at the top of his game. We'd hit the sauna, the jacuzzi, the pool and the restaurant. Everywhere he'd stop people: "This is my son. Teaches college up north." I'd quickly fill in my name. One club member praised an *LA Times* op-ed piece I had just written about Soviet Jews. The man's son, Daniel, would win a Pulitzer Prize for his book on the international oil crisis. I had far exceeded that pinnacle in my father's eyes with my freelance sports articles in *USA Today*. One morning I sat down to brunch at the Club with my father and Pete. We were an odd little trio. Here was Phil, back from the gambler's brink of despair, now working the other side of the street. He beamed as only the gainfully employed can.

"This is my boy," he told Pete. The latter, having returned that morning from Paris, looked like a washed out James Caan. He wore earthtones, tasseled taupe loafers and the requisite Rolex. Pete slid a bejeweled hand in my direction. We exchanged pleasantries. I had a ton of questions for him. How did you get started? What's your annual take? Ever been in prison? What's the biggest bet you ever covered? But I swallowed them all. None of us knew what to talk about. So we munched our bagels and sipped coffee. Later I asked my father what Pete reported as the source of his income. "He's partners in a pig farm in Acapulco."

Vegas was still the family destination of choice, although we no longer left at dawn in a '47 Oldsmobile. I joined my parents and brother Bill on one trip, our family of four taking advantage of a Vegas special—round trip flight from LA and a free meal at the casino for twenty bucks. Up and back in one day, enough to make you feel like a serious gambler.

The only stipulation was that you must gamble at least four hours with five dollar minimum bets. Plus, you must wear a tiny collar pin to identify you to casino officials. Was this the antithesis of Jews forced to wear the yellow Star of David? Anyone who wants to equate gambling with fate cannot ignore the facts. I could just as easily have been born in Europe in 1942, and experienced the hell of Hitler's Germany. But here I was in Benjamin Siegel's invention being identified by a lapel pin. Any way you want to look at it, fate deals each of us a hand. Some get annihilation, others a silver spoon. Or to quote Nick's sage father in *The Great Gatsby:* "A sense of the fundamental decencies is parceled out unequally at birth."

Looking back on it all, the odd thing is I thought nothing odd about this family. Gambling possessed each one of us, to varying degrees. I could never fathom my mother's take on gambling; she chastised my father when he lost, yet joined in as he indulged his addiction. She thought he had it under control, but my brother and I knew different. Bill often subsidized Dad's habit. What a family. On December 25 we celebrated not Christmas but the day before Opening Day at Santa Anita. When one of us returned from a vacation it wasn't "did you have a good time" but "how did you do?" When Dad went to work for Pete I got curious about Mom's reaction. "When you kids were little," she volunteered, "I wouldn't have let him do it." I assumed that she wouldn't have wanted her children stigmatized should their father end up in prison. After all, this would have been the 1950s, when even divorce was slightly scandalous.

My father may not have excelled in many of society's vaunted endeavors, but what a crap shooter! There were the three of us in Vegas—father and two sons—around the crap table. Bill and I continued to look less and less like brothers—he gained weight, lost hair and seemed not to care about his appearance. I had topped six feet sometime in my twenties, remained slim and tried to look stylish. But I could not compete with my father, who delighted in his Beverly Hills wardrobe.

When my father got the dice he was as smooth as Baryshnikov. He'd shake the two red cubes near his ear and fling them across the green felt. "Eleven," yelled the craps dealer. My father proceeded to make several more passes, each time stacking and unstacking chips, making numerous bets, his hands always in motion. He'd compute bets a step ahead of the dealers. (This man dropped out of high school?) "Press," he'd say often, doubling his bets.

Bill observed that when Dad had the hot hand he'd push it without fear. As for Bill himself, he admitted that "I play not to lose." Bill loved the action but with minimal risk. It was why he could set a loss limit and stop. For me, the ecstasy of winning was easily trumped by the anguish of losing. Of course, that truth wasn't enough to keep me out of the casino, especially since ecstasy was always a few quick passes away at the crap table. Once at Tahoe, in the days before ATMs, I was stuck several hundred when the dice caught fire. Within minutes I had struck for two thousand dollars. I walked to the cashier's window and bought back several checks I had written, gleefully tearing them to shreds. That's what keeps the chasers chasing—knowing how fast things can turn around.

Chapter 11

Gambler's Dream State

What non-gamblers do not know is the feeling of virtue—when the dice roll as one commands. And that omniscient goodness when the card you need rises to the top of the deck to greet your delighted yet confident eyes. It is as close as I have ever come in my life to a religious feeling.

—Mario Puzo

WHEN THE POLISH SOLIDARITY MOVEMENT STRUCK THE SHIPYARDS at Gdansk in the summer of 1980, I was sitting with my girlfriend Joanie in Venice watching the Gondolas glide past and trying to locate a casino. The two of us created a stir at the hotel front desk when Joanie asked the clerk if there was a casino nearby. "For him," the woman replied incredulously. "Yes," said Joanie. The staff members giggled. We quickly learned that "casino" was Italian for "brothel." We settled for Renaissance art (Joanie's passion) and saved the casino search for London.

"Try SoHo," suggested the Pakistani cab driver. So we did. The Charlie Chester Casino was at 12 Archer Street, a two-story affair with black marble walls, mirrored throughout. For five pounds you get a lifetime membership, which includes a booklet of 34 rules members must agree to. Rule number 8 states in part that "A member who parts with his membership card to a member of the public will be barred and shall forfeit all the privileges of memberships and all rights against the Company and the Club." Feeling very exclusive, Joanie and I climbed the stairs into the smoky den.

Here was the antithesis of Las Vegas. Charlie Chester's was family-owned, subdued save for an occasional loutish loser who found himself warned.

I transferred fifty pounds into chips and entered the gambler's dream state—a staggering lucky streak. The dice were firmly under my control; in fact, the whole table was hitting pass after pass. The owner turned slightly ashen as he watched the proceedings. The Brits were in awe of my run, cashing in right along with me. We raised the decibel level beyond what was proper. It was smoke and ale, good cheer and more British jokes about "forgiving our little Revolution" and the dice seemed devoid of sevens as I continued to hit point after point, taking the odds. Joanie stood behind me, enthralled. This oil well gushed for three straight days; even at the blackjack tables, upstairs, my luck prevailed.

When I contemplate the streak of my life, two decades later, oddly enough I cannot recall the amount I won—just that I had five- and ten-pound notes stuffed in every pocket. But I vividly recall a disquieting thought when it seemed that I couldn't lose. This is *too* good, *too* easy. I don't like it. My reaction was not unusual. Axel in James Toback's film *The Gambler* says that "if all my bets were safe, there just wouldn't be any juice." A similar sentiment was expressed by the George Siegel character in Robert Altman's film *California Split*.

What's going on? Isn't the giant score what it's all about? Mathematician Pascal, speaking of the gambler, put it bluntly:

"Give him the same amount of money every morning that he is likely to win during the day's play on condition that he does not gamble, and you will make him thoroughly unhappy. It will perhaps be said that he only cares about the fun of gambling and not his winnings. But make him play for nothing; he will not get any excitement out of it at all and will merely be bored. This means that he is not looking for entertainment alone. He must grow excited and fool himself into believing that he would be delighted to win the money that he would hate to be given to him on the condition that he does not gamble."

Chapter 12

The First Bet

Gambling is a questioning of Fortune. And the more she refuses to answer, the more we question. —André Suares

In the beginning, everything was even money. —Mike Caro

WHO MADE THE FIRST BET? Since Einstein says "God does not play dice," it must have been early man. That means for several millennia we have been a species addicted to risk. So when exactly did human beings discover this contradictory need to wager? Observes author Martin C. McGurrin:

Archaeologists have unearthed sufficient artifacts and documentation to establish certainly that human beings have wagered on the outcome of chance events for at least the past 6,000 years. Gambling is an ancient and universal human behavior. Some theorists speculate that its origins derive from the more occult aspects of early religious efforts to foretell the future, some suggest it was used cleverly by politicians and monarchs to distract the masses from the discomfort of food shortages or some other uncontrollable social calamity, and others regard gambling as a natural extension of play and recreation.

It is also certainly documented that, whatever the origins and broader social functions of gambling, with it came the problem, for some, of gambling uncontrollably. The inability to control the impulse to gamble and the continuation of wagering independent of the amount won or lost has an ancient record. Sooner or later, most human beings make a wager, but some of these persons do not attempt to stop wagering until their lives are in crisis as a consequence of their uncontrolled wagering.

No one can identify the first compulsive gambler. But centuries ago there were clearly some folks concerned about a popular vice that just might also be an illness.

Gerolamo Cardano seems the least likely candidate to succumb to gambling's scourge. A noted physician during Renaissance Italy, he wrote *The Book on Games of Chance* (circa 1530), the first study on the principles of probability. What's more, the work is peppered with sage observations on the gambler, including who should avoid gambling at his peril. "Gambling arouses anger and disturbs the mind," Cardano writes. "There must be moderation in the amount of money involved; otherwise, it is certain that no one should ever play."

Cardano's advice to those who believe gambling "relieves boredom" is almost comical for those addicts we find today welded to a slot machine. Imagine suggesting to a gambling compulsive that "your time will be better served by playing the lute, singing, or composing poetry."

Yet Cordano astutely says of the gambler:

If he is victorious, he wastes the money won by gambling; whereas if he suffers defeat, then either he is reduced to poverty, when he is honest and without resources or else to robbery, if he is powerful and dishonest; or again to the gallows, if he is poor and dishonest."

Cordano attacked the sad spectacle of "public gambling." (Governments did not run lotteries in those days.) "The most respectable place is at home or at the house of a friend, where there can be no public scandal."

Then a word to those of vaunted social status:

Lawyers, doctors and the like play at a disadvantage: for one thing, they appear to have too much leisure; for another, if they win, they seem to be gamblers, and if they lose, perhaps they may be taken to be as unskillful in their own art as in gaming.

He ends his thought with a nonsequitor: "Men of these professions incur the same judgment if they wish to practice music."

But Cordano was also intrigued with how character is forged by gambling:

Play is a very good test of a man's patience or impatience. The greatest advantage in gambling comes from not playing at all. But there is very great utility in it as a test of patience, for a good man will refrain from anger even at the moment of rising from the game in defeat.

Casino veterans of any era know that some rise from a shellacking with a good natured exit ("That's it, I'm tapped") while others toss the cards or pound the table in rage while giving the winners a stinging rebuke.

Before Cordano himself wound up destitute from gambling losses, he observed:

Even if gambling were altogether an evil, still, on account of the very large number of people who play, it would seem to be a natural evil. For that very reason it ought to be discussed by a medical doctor like one of the incurable diseases.

Cardano's wish that gambling be considered a medical problem was more than realized on November 7, 1834, when Charles Caldwell, MD, addressed medical students at Transylvania University, Lexington,

Kentucky, on "The Vice of Gambling." Professor Caldwell sought establishment of an Anti-Gambling Society endorsed by the officers and members of Transylvania University.

Caldwell's speech of more than 11,000 words was a genuine stemwinder—moralistic fervor, poignant examples, prescience and hyperbole unmatched by today's TV evangelists. Since he spoke at a time when gambling was in disrepute (there was a national clamor to ban lotteries) Caldwell confidently plunged into his talk with unrestrained bombast:

> I fearlessly assert, that a vice more nefarious in principle, more foul in its associations, more demoralizing in influence, or more destructive in its consequences, has scarcely an existence . . . For darkness of design, and depth of turpitude, intemperance (drinking), compared to it, is purity and innocence.

Caldwell alluded frequently to "recorded facts" that prove his conclusions, but he failed to cite them. However, he made several points that are the subject of gambling addiction research today, 170 years after his address.

On addiction:

> By being constantly and intensely exercised, the cerebral organs concerned in gambling attain a size and a degree of vigor, and are thrown into a state of excitement so inordinate, as to become ungovernable.

On predisposition:

> In many cases, the gambling monomania can be no more withstood, than that under which the invalid believes himself haunted by ghosts and goblins, visited by angels, or favoured by an intercourse with the apostles and prophets. But madness of every description is known to be communicable from parents to offspring . . . All accu-

rate observers and enlightened thinkers will acknowledge, that the gambling organs and propensity may become heirlooms in families, and thus the vice be perpetuated. . .

On destruction:

For every single instance of ruin and wretchedness arising from theft, pocket-picking, and robbery united, gambling alone produces thousands. Search the records of the four vices, written in despair, madness, suicide, bankruptcy, the reduction of wives and children from opulence and ease, to want and beggary, with their withered and tottering frames, sunken eyes, and squalid countenance, and the many other forms of individual, family, and social desolation thence resulting, and they will amply sustain the truth of my assertion.

Although melodramatic, Caldwell's assertions are currently supported by studies on gambling addiction as it relates to bankruptcies and suicide.

But when Caldwell does go over the top he leaves solid ground in great leaps:

[Gambling] is a native product of the human mind, rendered vicious by an ill-directed or a defective education, which has left certain animal propensities unsubdued, and neglected to strengthen the higher faculties, especially the moral and reflective one. Or the rebellious propensities may have been maddened and invigorated by profligate associates.

Caldwell then cites the mind's saving grace: "By persons, whose faculties are molded into a proper balance, by a thorough and sound education, gambling is never indulged in."

I must take issue with Caldwell on his point about "sound education." On more than one occasion I have heard Schopenhauer, and others of deep thought, discussed at the poker table.

Nor does the woman of the 1830s escape Caldwell's moral scalpel:

A passing notice of female gamblers may not be aimless for, disgraceful and offensive to delicacy as the fact is, society contains such unsexed beings. I have never known one of them that was an amiable woman. True; many amiable and estimable women, exemplary wives and excellent mothers, may be induced, to oblige others, to participate in what they consider the mere amusement of a card table.

But they never play to win, nor enter fiercely into the spirit of the game. Even in what they do, however, they act improperly, by setting an example to their families, they may prove disastrous. But, different from these, as vice is from virtue, ferocity from mildness, and impudence from modesty, are female gamblers. They engage in the sport with inordinate devotedness, play furiously for gain, and are, without an exception, shrews and termagants. Were they not so, they would have neither taste nor fitness for the game. And, to their other exceptional qualities, they usually add the more petty, but hardly less disreputable vices of tattling, slander, and unladylike languages.

Shrews and termagants? Dr. Caldwell meet Annie Duke, mother of four, Ivy League grad, and one of the world's top ten poker players. Duke won close to $150,000 at the annual Las Vegas World Series of Poker in 2003. She says her life competing on the professional poker circuit is "the perfect job for a mom." And, she explains, "if I have a sick child or a soccer game, I don't have to play." ("Of course," I can hear Dr. Caldwell piping up, "but what about all the mothers addicted to poker without Annie Duke's skill?")

Surely some of Caldwell's assertions must have drawn titters from the students, such as:

> The vice [the gambler] has contracted, sordid in its nature, and as rank in venom as the 'plague of leprosy,' clings to his reputation, like the tunic to Hercules, and infects it with a malady, as deep and incurable, as it is foul and repulsive.

Caldwell concludes with a futile gesture against the Sport of Kings, horse racing. Surely he was aware that Lexington prided itself on its lush thoroughbred breeding farms. Or maybe not. "For one form of gambling," he says, "which is alarmingly fashionable, a more plausible defence is attempted. I anticipate, therefore, some difficulty in convincing even pure minded men, and deliberate thinkers, who have not thoroughly examined the subject, that the sport is vicious, and the defence of it fallacious . . . It may scarcely be added, I allude to horse-racing."

Caldwell becomes positively Shakespearean in his range of imagery:

> When we look on the crowd that assembles to witness the scene, listen to their licentious and profane discourse, examine their wild bacchanalian carousals, observe their reckless dissipation of means, which they ought to appropriate to better purposes, and reflect on the consequences, our sentiments change. We almost sicken at the contrast, are ready to denounce the spectacle as infamous, and to proclaim the horses by far more worthy and honorable animals, than most of the human beings around them.

Caldwell might have been dismayed to learn that four decades later, in 1875, roughly 70 miles to the west of Lexington, in Louisville, the Kentucky Derby was launched and remains the most famous horse race in the United States. It has been held the first Saturday in May of every year since, featuring a subdued "bacchanalian spectacle" of mint juleps and a tearful group rendition of "My Old Kentucky Home." No less an official personage than the governor of Kentucky presents the winner's trophy.

Caldwell got full support for his Anti-Gambling Society of Transylvania University, complete with a constitution, which notes in article 3:

> The members of the Society, on signing this Constitution, pledge themselves to abstain from every species of betting, and all kinds of games of chance for money or property, and in every proper and honorable way to discourage and suppress the vice of gambling.

Surely a game, but losing, effort.

An equally powerful voice against gambling appeared ten years later, in 1844, with the publication of Jonathan H. Green's memoir, *Gambling Unmasked*. Green's tale reads like *Candide* meets Damon Runyon. The author is battered from one revolting gambling scene to the next, from callow youth to adulthood.

The purpose of his book is "to warn the young of the snares and temptations that beset their path. [Green] shows, that the lures to gaming are numerous; that in all its forms it is a scheme to defraud; that it is never an innocent amusement, for even in its incipient stages it is associated with or leads to guilt, and if persisted in tends to irretrievable ruin."

Gambling Unmasked was plucked from obscurity in 2000 by *The Wager* *(Weekly Addiction Gambling Education Report)* of the Division on Addictions at Harvard Medical School. *The Wager* posed the question: "Would the J. H. Green of the early 19th century be considered a pathological gambler by standards drafted in the late 20th century?" It applied criteria from the American Psychiatric Association's *Diagnostic and Statistical Manual of Mental Disorders (DSM-IV)* of 1980, which classified pathological gambling as an impulse control disorder and considered anyone meeting at least five of the ten criteria to be a pathological gambler.

Green's narrative: I had abandoned all hope . . . The force of evil habit, and the accumulation of guilt, seemed too great to throw off; and the prospect of reformation . . . seemed to be to be gone forever.

DSM-IV symptom: Has repeated unsuccessful efforts to control, cut back, or stop gambling.

Green's narrative: . . . yielding to the solicitations of the gambler added to my grief, yet I still kept up appearances, and that too at the expense of my acquaintances.

DSM-IV symptom: . . . has jeopardized or lost a significant relationship, job, or educational or career opportunity because of gambling.

Green's narrative: I counted my money over and over, and never expected to play anymore. The whole live-long night I was troubled by the excitement of the faro bank.

DSM-IV symptom: . . . is restless or irritable when attempting to cut down or stop gambling.

Green's narrative: Yet the deep and abiding anxiety I had to see my father, and to enjoy his society once more, made me lose all control over myself, and my interest had to give way to my passion.

DSM-IV symptom: . . . gambles as a way of escaping from problems or relieving a dysphoric mood (e.g., feelings of helplessness, guilt, anxiety, depression).

The Wager found that Green had four of the DSM-IV symptoms, rendering him ineligible for a diagnosis of pathological gambling, but still a problem gambler.

While the US was suffering the effects of a bitter Civil War (during which soldiers on both sides gambled at cards even as battles raged) the great Russian novelist Fyodor Dostoyevsky was taking a month off from work on his masterpiece, *Crime and Punishment*. In a flurry he wrote *The Gambler* (1866), an astute psychological portrait of one Alexey Ivanovitch. Dostoyevsky's own gambling addiction was well known; *The Gambler* would later provide fodder for Freud and his contemporaries to mull over in great depth.

Along with intrigue, suspense and betrayal, *The Gambler* reveals much of the protagonist's psyche. Alexey admits that "even on my way to the gambling hall, as soon as I hear, two rooms away, the clink of the scattered money I almost go into convulsions." And also his reed-thin rationale for gambling: "I had the strange and mad idea that I should be sure to win here at the gambling table. Why I had the idea I can't understand, but I believed in it. Who knows, perhaps I believed it because no other alternative was left me."

Dostoyevsky "invented" the plot line for *The Gambler* as he himself wagered ruble after ruble on a roulette system that brought him to the edge of financial ruin. "The main thing," the author wrote about his hero in *The Gambler,* "is that all his vital sap, his energies, rebellion, daring, have been channeled into roulette. He is a gambler, and not merely an ordinary gambler . . . He is a poet in his own way, but the fact is that he himself is ashamed of the poetic element in him, because deep down he feels it is despicable . . . the need to take risks ennobles him in his own eyes."

As for the force of the book itself, take one master novelist, imbue him with a severe gambling habit, and the result on the page is almost inevitable. Observes Joseph Frank in *Dostoyevsky: The Miraculous Years, 1865-71*: "The gambling scenes are in a class by themselves, and no one, before or since, has depicted the intoxicating delirium of a gambling obsession with such intimate mastery."

Chapter 13

Norman R et al.

*The race is not always to the swift nor the battle to the strong. But that's
the way to bet.*

                                        —Damon Runyan

MY OWN LIFE WASN'T QUITE AS SWEET AS MY FATHER'S during the start of his
bookie days. I was enduring staggering losses at Lake Tahoe. They were
covered by my paychecks—I had few expenses—but the repeated blows to
the ego were not. The drive home through colossal mountains on narrow,
icy roads seemed wrong for someone in rank depression. I once contemplated a plunge to oblivion. Reno was a much safer destination, a straight
shot up highway 80.

Along with gambling binges and journalism teaching, I also wrote
freelance feature stories for local newspapers and magazines. Naturally,
I gravitated toward pieces on gambling. One article for the *San Francisco
Examiner* got me up in the announcer's booth at Golden Gate Fields,
profiling the race caller. I had to crawl across the roof and squeeze into
the tiny cubicle. But it was a thrill to look down at the brown oval track,
colorful jockeys on their mounts, the crowd floating here and there like
amoebas under a microscope. The race caller, John Gibson, answered a
question that had always plagued me—how can you tell which horse is

which? "Don't memorize the horses and the numbers," he said. "It's a trap." The secret was to memorize horse and silks color, since the numbers on the saddles can get blocked from view.

I wrote a first-person account for the *Oakland Tribune* in 1990 about playing in a poker tournament. I lost $250, but pocketed $100 for the piece. I came in 12th, five places out of the money.

My story started:

> Who says there's no such thing as a free lunch? I had one at the Oaks Club in Emeryville that cost me $250. The free lunch came with entering the Oaks Club Hold 'Em Poker Tournament.
>
> Why was I there? Just as the sandlot baseball player dreams of cracking a World Series homer and the weekend tennis player fantasizes Centre Court at Wimbledon, social card players also have their dreams. Mine was bumping heads with real poker talent.

My most emotional freelance writing experience was a topic I could no longer avoid—Gamblers Anonymous. First I did my homework.

Jim W. founded Gamblers Anonymous in 1957. Jim was no bookish dilettante; he gambled himself into despair and landed in Alcoholics Anonymous. That was a blessing. Jim took AA's principles and applied them to gambling. He knew the therapeutic value of talking about his addiction and meeting with others so afflicted.

Jim modeled GA on the principles of Alcoholics Anonymous, utilizing the AA 12-step program. Compulsive gamblers talk about their addiction ("giving testimony") and often come to realize they are helpless unless they achieve total abstinence.

Since Jim's death in 1983 Gamblers Anonymous chapters have kept pace with the prevalence of legalized gambling, more than doubling from 650 chapters in 1990 to 1328 in 1998. GA success is hard to measure; clients maintain anonymity and few records are kept. Anecdotal evidence of abstention abounds; but there is no way of knowing how many attend a few GA meetings and return to the world of addiction. In fact, the only known survey on the effectiveness of GA, according the *National Gambling Impact Study Report,* found that "only 8 percent of GA members were in abstinence after one year in the group." And yet, every gambling treatment specialist I contacted spoke highly of GA. The recognition that others share the addiction is a powerful tonic for some compulsive gamblers. They are, in effect, detoxing their shame.

I attended GA meetings in San Francisco and Oakland resulting in a magazine piece in 1985. The meetings were painful, liberating, instructive. I had come face to face with cautionary tales, told by survivors who acknowledged that the hellish demon is always one bet away. I readily agreed to change names and mask identities. The classic writer's advice to "empathize with your subject" was never easier.

My article, titled "Gamblers Anonymous: Last Exit on the Highway to Hell," opened with one man's plight:

> Norman R. was face down in a drunk tank when he had a revelation: "Stop gambling or die." He stopped. That was seven years ago. Norman keeps the gambling demons in check by telling his horror stories over and over again at Gamblers Anonymous meetings.

Some members attend three meetings a week, finding it valuable to talk about the addiction and to hear others in similar pain. Carl, for example, spent years denying his addiction. "I'd leave the casino with a wrenched feeling in my gut," he said. "And incredible guilt. I'd lose the rent money. The food money. Then I'd be back gambling the next day. I knew I couldn't continue to live my life this way."

Martin was making his fifth attempt at GA. He scrapped plans for a vacation to the Bahamas when he found himself plotting ways to bring extra money and then sneak off the beach to the casino. He told his GA brethren: "I knew if I did that I couldn't face you guys."

A watershed event in the treatment of compulsive gamblers took place in 1972 at the VA Hospital in Brecksville, Ohio, where Dr. Robert Custer established the first inpatient treatment center. Often referred to as "the father of professional help for the compulsive gambler," Custer was co-founder of the National Council on Compulsive Gambling and spearheaded the effort to get compulsive gambling classified as a psychiatric disorder by the American Psychiatric Association. His book, *When Luck Runs Out: Help for Compulsive Gamblers and Their Families* (1984), was read widely by practitioners and those afflicted with gambling addiction.

In the early 1970s, Custer was mute on the topic of compulsive gambling. "Although I had done some thinking about the subject of compulsive gambling and had heard it discussed once or twice at psychiatric meetings," Custer wrote, "I had never had occasion to treat a patient with this disorder and would not have known where to begin if someone with that ailment came in and asked for help. I knew only about the psychoanalytic approach, which held that compulsive gamblers are masochists and need to undergo psychoanalytic treatment to relieve their guilt and their supposed need to be punished. I do not hold with this view. To me, compulsive gambling appeared to be a disorder of impulse control. . ."

Custer attended several GA meetings. Experienced in treating alcoholics, Custer "was prepared for similarities." But what struck him after just a GA meeting or two "was not just the similarity in the programs but the similarity between the people—the compulsive gamblers and the alcoholics—and between the two disorders—compulsive gambling and alcoholism. This came as a big surprise, because I could not see how there could possibly be any relationship between an addiction to a drug and a behavioral problem like compulsive gambling. Nevertheless, the similarities were there." Custer was prescient, for two decades later compulsive gambling would be labeled the "invisible addiction." Custer was instrumental in getting the American Psychiatric Association to list Compulsive Gambling as an "impulse control disorder" in the 1980 update of the *Diagnostic Statistical Manual* (DSM-III).

Not everyone agrees that compulsive gambling is, in fact, an "impulse control disorder." In their article "Refuting the Myths of Compulsive Gambling," Richard E. Vatz and Lee S. Weinberg start by considering some high-profile cases of compulsive gamblers. Their most notable celebrity gambler is Pete Rose, the major league baseball player who was banned for life from the sport:

> In mid-1989, it was revealed that baseball hero Pete Rose had dropped more than $500,000 through heavy gambling. It was also reported that he had to sell treasured memorabilia because of his debts. After weeks of bad press following a denial that he had a problem with gambling, Rose made a public statement that he had what his recently acquired psychiatrist called a "clinically significant gambling disorder" that rendered him powerless over his gambling. He then went on a media tour, during which he was greeted by a lengthy standing ovation from Phil Donahue's television audience and congratulations for his "admission" from Barbara Walters. Rose had gone from miscreant to courageous victim. [Fifteen years later, 2004, Rose would finally admit publicly having bet on baseball and publish *My Prison Without Bars* in his long shot bid for admission to the Baseball Hall of Fame.]

"The problem is that there is no evidence that compulsive gambling is a disease," the authors write. Worse, they conclude, "the consequences of accepting compulsive gambling as addictive or uncontrollable may be to hinder efforts of heavy gamblers to resist their urges."

Vatz and Weinberg make a compelling case, certainly one that most relatives of compulsive gamblers would be eager to accept. The authors refute the authorities' claim of gambling "addiction" step by step, even seizing on a quote from the president of the National Council on Problem Gambling, Sirgay Sanger, in the Journal of the American Medical Association: "Pathological gambling 'has the smell of a biochemical addiction in it,' but, he admits, 'there is no research proof.'"

The authors go on to compare gambling to other addictions:

The debate about compulsive gambling like that about other self-destructive or socially unacceptable behaviors ranging from compulsive drinking to compulsive shopping (a supposed new disorder whose advocates urge its inclusion in the next revision of psychiatry's diagnostic manual), ultimately comes down to a single question: Should individuals who engage in these behaviors be excused on the grounds that they suffer from a disorder that produces urges they are unable to resist? Without further evidence, we believe that the answer to be no.

Since the authors offered their views in 1993, I contacted Vatz, a professor of rhetoric and communication, a decade later to see if current research had altered his view. "Not at all," he said immediately. "If anything, I feel stronger about it." Vatz holds to his concluding statement condemning the medical community: "This much is clear: it is time to stop all special consideration for those whose excuses are sympathy-provoking only because they bear the unscientific 'disorder' imprimatur of psychiatry."

Vatz's words did not shake my belief in the impulse control disorder theory. But they did spark an image of a compulsive gambler riding the thrill of casino action. He's on a horrid losing streak. "You know," his inner voice says, "you can stop any time." The thought registers, but the gambler is imprisoned in the present and cannot—or will not—concede the existence of tomorrow.

I wrote several more GA articles, always leaving the intense sessions with three words stitched before my eyes: You've Been Warned. Result: I became the equivalent of a binge eater—a binge gambler. I'd cross the line into addiction, the pain palpable, then return to a life of teaching. I rarely dealt in introspection. But after several days "clean" I could hear the shrill call of the dice. And I'd gas up on the weekend and head for that slice of

Nevada just across the California line. If I permitted myself an honest reckoning it would be this: I beat the casinos rarely, perhaps once in ten trips.

I shared my secret life with a Laney College math professor, Noah, whose own father had worked the rackets in New York and ended up in a long prison stretch. Noah wasn't as sanguine about his father as I was about mine. In fact, Noah became a bearded Marxist and shunned contact with his father.

Noah asked if I would like to give a guest lecture on "dice and probability" to his algebra class. The thought got my juices churning. Just preparing the lecture felt like a walk into the casino, my brain buzzing with anticipation. After a near sleepless night, I downed several cups of coffee. Totally wired, I entered the classroom bearing a pair of red Vegas dice. I scribbled the 36 dice combinations on the board:

1 + 1 = 2	2 + 1 = 3	3 + 1 = 4	4 + 1 = 5	5 + 1 = 6	6 + 1 = 7
1 + 2 = 3	2 + 2 = 4	3 + 2 = 5	4 + 2 = 6	5 + 2 = 7	6 + 2 = 8
1 + 3 = 4	2 + 3 = 5	3 + 3 = 6	4 + 3 = 7	5 + 3 = 8	6 + 3 = 9
1 + 4 = 5	2 + 4 = 6	3 + 4 = 7	4 + 4 = 8	5 + 4 = 9	6 + 4 = 10
1 + 5 = 6	2 + 5 = 7	3 + 5 = 8	4 + 5 = 9	5 + 5 = 10	6 + 5 = 11
1 + 6 = 7	2 + 6 = 8	3 + 6 = 9	4 + 6 = 10	5 + 6 = 11	6 + 6 = 12

I felt exalted. Here I was, another Moses, or Elmer Gantry, about to share something essential, divine! After a brief disclaimer about how I was not advocating gambling, blah blah blah, I put the question to them: If I were to throw these dice, which number would be the most logical for you to bet on?

"Ten," yelled one student.

"Why?"

"It's my lucky number." Laughter.

I put it in terms of probability. "Which number is most likely to turn up?"

Stunned silence. "What about two or twelve," I said, circling the first and last combinations. A student up front noted that there is only one way to make each combination. "Right," I said. "The odds against making either 2 (Snake eyes) or 12 (Boxcars) are 35 to 1." Heads nodded. I was getting jazzed. "Now, which number has the most combinations?" More silence. I circled the six combinations that make seven. Several noted the pattern on the board. I explained that once one die is thrown, no matter what it lands on, you can still make a seven. But that was not true of any other number. I was elated. Some found this dreary; but several students were tuning in. "So," I proceeded, "what are the odds of making a seven on one roll of the dice?"

"Six to one," said a voice from the back.

"Close," I said. "The chances are one in six but the odds are five to one." Several people were anxious for me to throw the dice. One young man wanted to know the rules of dice. Several students egged me on.

I glanced at Noah; he nodded okay. Just as I was explaining the pass line and taking the odds, a college administrator stuck his head into the classroom. I returned to probability. "Remember," I stressed, "just because seven is the most likely number to come up doesn't mean it will. In fact, there are thirty other combinations, so the chances are it will not be a seven." I reminded them that probability is merely a predictor of what may happen. Not what will happen. "There is nothing stopping me from throwing twelves all day."

"Would you bet on that happening?" someone asked.

"Not with your money."

Now they were primed. Several students yelled out their numbers. I tossed the dice the length of the table, watching them bounce off the chalkboard and clack-clack as they came to rest on the table. I waited while the suspense built. "Nine," I shouted to scattered cheers. My pulse raced; it was as if I had just left a winning session at the crap table. Noah was later reprimanded for my "gambling" talk. He was amused—and also tenured. Talking passionately about gambling seemed to satisfy some level

of my craving for casino action. It hadn't occurred to me then that scour-
ing gambling addiction literature might have the same salutary effect.

The next few years are fluid in my memory—gambling despite myself,
visits to my folks in LA and attending the High Sierra's Super Bowl of
Poker, Lake Tahoe's answer to the annual World Series of Poker in Las
Vegas. I managed a writing assignment in the mid-1980s for *USA Today*,
exulting in a chance to be up close with the world's top poker players.

The rules are the same as in Vegas: anyone can enter by merely plunk-
ing down $10,000. No more buy-ins; the field plays until someone has all
the chips. The game is no limit Texas Hold 'Em, with each player dealt
two cards down while five "communal cards" are turned up in the middle
of the table, first three (the "flop") then a fourth (the "turn") and fifth
(the "river"). There are four rounds of betting. Bluffing is at a premium.
In fact, I once watched the late wispy Stu Ungar shove $300,000 into the
pot. His opponent nearly swallowed his Stetson, folding meekly. Ungar
uncharacteristically flashed a hole card, revealing that he was on a bust
hand (bluffing).

The Super Bowl winner gets 50 percent of the total take. These are not
compulsive gamblers, of course. They are pro gamblers who differ mark-
edly from the addicted—they have skill, discipline and the ability to walk
away from a disastrous run at the table. Some compulsives have the illusion they are pros in training, convinced of their skill but merely having
a run of bad luck. It's a sad revelation when—and if—they face the truth.
But the pro gamblers are also a quirky lot, some sporting giant Stetsons,
others with dark glasses to conceal "tells," yet others with Mafia-style
rings jammed onto several fingers. The legendary, dapper Amarillo Slim
was the Super Bowl of Poker "host," commentating when the play was
down to the final seven players and the TV cameras moved in.

The final winning hand was a lowly pair of eights, held by Mickey
Appleman, who had an MBA from Ohio State University and described
himself as "a sports handicapper." He pocketed $205,000. One reporter

was foolish enough to ask Appleman what he was going to do with the money. Appleman shot him a sour glance: "The game's never over." Appleman is quoted in *The Biggest Game in Town,* A. Alvarez's homage to the rarefied world of the poker masters. "Gambling helped me more than analysis," Appleman says. "I suffered from depression—I was so entwined with my inner world I never had a chance to enjoy myself. For me, activity was the answer. I took up gambling after I finished with psychoanalysis, and the depression never returned."

Gamblers without Appleman's proven skills are advised against such therapy.

Chapter 14

The Longest Walk

It's a terrible feeling to be far ahead and then start losing in a way that you just can't stop. There comes a point when you begin to think you know the cards before they're dealt.

—Frederick and Steven Barthelme

My Vegas visits over several decades have blended into a pattern of dashed hopes. Yet, my most painful sojourn did not involve financial loss. I had met my parents in Vegas for their wedding anniversary (an annual pilgrimage). We were all booked into downtown hotels, my parents at the Union Plaza and I at the other end of then-seamy Fremont Street.

Our family rite of passage was hitting the royal flush on the 25 cent poker machine—always playing five coins to insure a payoff of at least $1000. I hit my first at Circus Circus on The Strip, catching the ten-and-queen of clubs to the jack, king, ace. Bells rang. People screamed. My pulse quickened. Before they could count out my $1100 winnings my father was already whispering in my ear: "I'd put the touch on you but your mother would kill me." I took my cue: "But how would she find out?" I slipped my father $300. Since I was already stuck two hundred for the trip, my winnings were now six hundred. I vowed that "just this once, I'm going to leave Vegas a winner."

That night as a "winner" I walked the longest block of my life—downtown Fremont Street. I only had to pass seven or eight hotels to reach mine. But the hotels' casino entrances are on the sidewalk, emitting slot machine bells and winners' screams, with pitchmen outside enticing passersby. I strode into one hotel and lost $200 without winning one bet. I downed two beers and floated into the next place. Craps and blackjack both produced uncommonly bad hands; not even a brief winning run. A clear message—stop. But I easily rationalized that I was not really losing money. These were winnings. My vow wasn't as potent as when I made it, but I still clung to my promise to leave town a winner. More free beer. My feet felt heavy as I trudged into the August evening heat, then back into the air-conditioned casinos.

In my alcoholic stupor, I was both jinxed and challenged. When my stake dropped below $300 I felt the anger and helplessness of a loser. Stop, I told myself. Settle for a win of three hundred. Stop! But I couldn't. All gambling addicts know the feeling—total jinx. Practically every bet a loser. A twenty at the blackjack table means nothing even if the dealer's showing garbage. She'll hit that sixteen with a five—you know it in your gut. But you keep betting. My anger turned to silent rage. Muscles tightened, I could feel it in my neck and shoulders.

Several more beers left me weaving along Fremont Street, the experience surreal, an alcoholic shield blunting reality. Still, I felt cursed—but could not stop. I changed a twenty into quarters and played the poker machine, a change of pace. Perhaps I'd hit another royal flush, pick up $1,000, a new stake. Then I could face the crap table with a cushion, run this disaster into a happy ending. The poker machine sucked up the coins. Zip. Nada. Zilch.

Finally I reached my own hotel's casino. The jinx was waiting for me. Yet, I could not stop gambling. Finally I bet the last twenty dollars at blackjack, getting 19. The dealer hit a sixteen—pulling a four. As the dealer's winning card hit the green felt table I felt its full force, a body blow that left me limp. Suddenly sober, I contemplated chasing the six hundred dollars but knew that actually coming out a loser on this trip would leave me in a state of unmanageable despair.

I walked glumly to the elevator, then across the hall carpet to my room, into the all-mirrored bathroom where I faced a dilemma: how was I going to brush my teeth without looking at myself?

A few weeks after my Fremont Street walk of shame, I was in my journalist persona covering a GA meeting. At its conclusion I was asked if I had anything I'd like to say. "Yes," I was surprised to hear myself respond. And I told about my Vegas vow and the long walk down Fremont Street and the drinking and the turmoil and the jinx. When I explained my dilemma in the all-mirrored bathroom I saw that each GA member around the table was nodding in recognition.

Years later they would turn the semi-sleazy area, long known as "Glitter Gulch," into "The Fremont Experience," blocks and blocks of kiosks and souvenir hawkers and musicians and a psychedelic light show projected on the ceiling featuring, among others, the Beatles and Rolling Stones. At one of the latter, guitars rev to full blast while Mick Jagger's signature tongue seems large enough to lick the sky—downtown Las Vegas's answer to the seduction of The Strip.

Chapter 15

An Encore for Pete

The cops had a rap sheet on my father, including license plates, everything he had been doing.

MY FATHER QUIT PETE THE BOOKIE AFTER A FIVE-YEAR RUN. But he agreed to stay on a few days to train the new man. The new man was astounded to see my father writing 100 tickets a day. The novice was soon on his own, but the police nailed him within a month on the job, ending his employment.

So Pete asked my father to come back to work at $500 a week. By this time my parents were living in Marina del Rey, planning a move to a retirement community north of San Diego. But they agreed to one more year for Pete. My father drives out to the new apartment on San Vicente. "My first day back on the job," my father says with a mixture of shock and amusement, "the cops break down the door and arrest me." The cops had apparently been watching him all those years. "Hey Phil," they said. "How ya doin'?" The cops had a rap sheet on my father, including license plates, everything he had been doing. No one found out why the cops hadn't moved on my father sooner. Perhaps they were after Pete, the bigger fish.

My father admits, "I was glad it was the police." It could have been armed thugs with the mistaken impression that my father had wads of cash lying around. "I knew I would get caught eventually," he says. "It was the law of averages." My father was promptly taken off to jail in Culver City. He spent about five hours in a cell. He phoned my mother, who phoned Pete, who bailed him out. A court date was set.

My father relates his day in court in his inimitable style. "Pete gets me this lawyer and I meet him at the courthouse, in West LA. I don't know him right off from Pete's description but I recognize him by his fancy briefcase. My attorney goes up to the judge. They're telling jokes to each other! They're laughing, having a ball. The courthouse is full. Judge nods to him a couple of times. Attorney comes back to me. Says 'When he calls your name all you have to do is raise your hand.'" Pete took care of the fine. But my father knew his bookmaking days were over. The judge's advice was unambiguous: "Stop."

Chapter 16

Pure and Hidden

Winning money in a casino is really an attempt to alleviate the bank-ruptcy of the soul. —Dr. Paul Good

THE GAMBLING LITERATURE HAS MOVED BEYOND THE "DISEASE THEORIES" of Drs. Cordano and Caldwell, the "psychic masochism" of Dr. Bergler and the "infantile regression" of Freud and Simmel. But the American Psychiatric Association's "impulse control disorder" theory remains current as researchers try to understand why some people have no control over such destructive impulses.

Compulsive gambling research started to attract major grants in the 1990s. It attained a new status, writes researcher David E. Comings: "Pathological gambling has been termed both the 'pure' and the 'hidden' addiction. 'Pure' because it is not associated with the intake of any addicting substance, and 'hidden' because it is an extension of a common, socially accepted behavior."

Researchers seeking the ultimate cause of pathological gambling have some prime targets: genetics, chemical reactions in the brain and "co-morbidity" (linking gambling to other addictions). Recent research papers have such exotic titles as "A study of the dopamine D^2 receptor gene in patho-logical gambling," "The Molecular Genetics of Pathological Gambling," and "Familial influences on gambling behavior: an analysis of 3359 twin pairs."

Much of this research has found its way into the mainstream media—in translation. For example, it means little to most of us to learn that dopa-mine is "a monoamine C^8H11NO^2 that is a decarboxylated form of dopa and that occurs especially as a neurotransmitter in the brain." But when we read in the *San Francisco Chronicle* (May 28, 2001) that "scientists don't need to visit crowded casinos to prove that people get high on gambling" our layman's interest has been piqued. Further, says neuroscientist Dr. Hans Breiter, "We cannot distinguish any difference between the brain pat-tern of someone while gambling or ingesting cocaine." Dopamine, it turns out, is the "feel good" chemical that signals the brain "More! More."

But to get that "hit," the dopamine "receptor" (a protein on the surface of the brain cell) must interact with the dopamine gene. Comings found that 50 percent of pathological gamblers lacked the beneficial receptor gene and therefore experienced a shortage of dopamine's feel-good mes-sage. "Gamblers with this genetic variation may suffer from a chronic deprivation of dopamine. Gamblers may not be satisfied with the normal rewards. To compensate for the dopamine deficit, the person turns to activities that provide a jolt of dopamine. That rush keeps the gamblers coming back again and again to the blackjack table or some other game."

Brain circuitry research started to heat up in 2000. "Most of our daily deci-sions are just unconscious reactions," according to a *New York Times* article (February 19, 2002) quoting neuroscientist P. Read Montague, who estimates "that 90 percent of what people do every day is carried out by this kind of automatic, unconscious system that evolved to help creatures survive."

Animals use these circuits to know what to attend to, what to ignore and what is worth learning about. People use them for the same purposes which, as a result of their bigger brains and culture, include listening to music, eating chocolate, assessing beauty, gambling, investing in stocks and experimenting with drugs—all topics that have been studied this past year with brain imaging machines that direct the activity of human brain circuits.

For the pathological gambler concerned with what dopamine might be doing to his life, there is this: "The number of things people do to increase their dopamine firing rates is unlimited . . . Several studies were published last year (2001) looking at monetary rewards and dopamine. Money is abstract, but to the brain it looks like cocaine, food, sex, or anything a person expects is rewarding," said Dr. Beiter, a neuroscientist at Harvard, in the same *Times* article. "People crave it."

Our ancestors who were hunters and gatherers may now be at the dice table, hunting for that winning toss which, unconsciously, produces a thrilling blast of dopamine. This could involve many rolls of the dice and, in extreme cases of "bad luck," lead to the dissolution of a marriage. Or worse.

Always peeking over my shoulder, of course, is Professor Vatz, who would most likely put dopamine in the same category with the "impulse control disorder," as a medical excuse for letting the compulsive gambler off the hook. Can't personal responsibility override all this unconscious brain activity?

Slogging through tomes of footnote-laden gambling research for the non-scientist such as myself must be like a scientist trying to grasp the minutia of the *Daily Racing Form*. The compulsive gambler seeks to divine the winner; the researcher seeks the key to the gambler's passion. Following are conclusions of recent research (with sources at the end of the chapter):

• Gamblers reach an aroused, euphoric state comparable to the "high" derived from cocaine or other drugs, the presence of cravings, the development of tolerance (increasingly larger bets or greater risks needed to produce a desired level of excitement) and the experience of withdrawal-like symptoms (1)

• The anticipation of the big win releases a rush of feel-good chemicals in the brain. The gambler may be hooked, not on cocaine or another illicit drug, but on natural substances made by the body. (2)

• There is a typical course of progression in compulsive gambling through four stages—winning, losing, desperation, and hopelessness. (3)

• As with most addictions, the common perception is that people should be able to control their involvement and those who overindulge have only themselves to blame. While it is important for individuals to take responsibility for their own behavior, it is equally clear that biological and genetic factors can play a role in increasing the risk of becoming a pathological gambler. (4)

• Familial factors—inheritance and/or experiences shared by twin siblings during childhood—explain a substantial portion of the risk for pathological gambling behavior and for symptoms and diagnosis of pathological gambling disorder. (5)

• Alcoholism is relatively common among gamblers in treatment and co-occurs with pathological gambling in population-based epidemiological studies. The prevalence of pathological gambling is also increased among alcoholics in treatment. Illicit substance abuse and pathological gambling often overlap. (6)

So what does a clinician do with all this data? Put another way, how does today's therapist treat the compulsive gambler? A leading researcher, Richard R. Rosenthal, MD, has one foot in several of the above studies and another in what he calls the "psychodynamic approach" to the treatment of pathological gambling.

Rosenthal is convinced that pathological gamblers can achieve abstinence, which is essential if they acknowledge their addiction and assume responsibility in their treatment. To bring this about, the clinician becomes "a therapeutic ally by stimulating the patient's curiosity about the meaning and consequences of his behavior." But Rosenthal recognizes several roadblocks:

> The very fact of the patient coming for treatment more often than not represents an enormous failure for them. Some were coerced or blackmailed into it. Others, although propelled by inner pain or the desperation of their situation, had second thoughts immediately upon making the appointment. They feel guilty and ashamed, and while one might not always empathize with their discomfort (they are often very good at masking it), the very fact that they need help is evidence of their humiliation.

And then there is the pathological gambler's frequent ambivalence about treatment: Citing researcher J. I. Taber, Rosenthal explains:

> On the one hand, patients fear treatment will turn out to be just one more failure in their lives. At the same time, they fear its success, that deceptions will be unmasked, changes imposed on them, and that they will have to give up the one comfort in their lives, their gambling.

These fears surely kept my father from seeking help during his dog days of gambling addiction. "Successful treatment equals no more gambling," I can hear his psyche moan.

How does the compulsive gambler explain his addiction? Rosenthal's research led him to six discrete reasons:

(1) *Need for spectacular success.* "It is based on the need to demonstrate one's worth and get the approval of others."

(2) *Rebelliousness and anger.* "Such gambling is a way to thumb their noses or in fantasy punish the other. This is partly based on an

assumption of gambling as deviant behavior, which they know their families and others look down upon.

(3) *Freedom from dependency.* "People who feel overly dependent, for approval or validation from others, look for substitute activities and objects which they can control. Despite its reputation for risk-taking, gambling is a rather predictable activity."

(4) *Social acceptance.* "Many gamblers mention the perks they received, and how important it was that the various casino employees remembered their name, lit their cigarette, or brought them a drink. They felt accepted and valued."

(5) *Escape from painful or intolerable thoughts.* "This is the self-medication hypothesis . . . When people who are depressed gamble, they may experience an increase in energy, or a release of endorphins . . . there seems to be a temporary antidepressant effect."

(6) *Competitiveness.* "Many of the gamblers grew up feeling unappreciated and neglected by their families. There was a need to excel in order to get attention . . . Perseverance was particularly valued, although this same trait would later get them in trouble, when they would chase gambling losses."

Of course, most problem gamblers never get into treatment and so are not forced to peer beyond the surface of their reason for gambling. "I simply enjoy it," as my father would say. On my odyssey, I ponder my father's total lack of reflection on his addiction. Then I recall his reaction to an article I wrote on Gamblers Anonymous, filled with horrid tales. I mailed him a copy. Eagerly anticipating praise, I phoned him after a decent interval. "Didn't read it," he said simply.

When it comes to "chasing," the downfall of many a gambler, Rosenthal's insight seems especially acute: "During the course of the disorder they become increasingly intolerant of losses, and as shame, guilt, and depression worsen, they are increasingly desperate to win back what they lost. They take greater risks, abandon any reasonable gambling strategies, and become increasingly irrational in their thinking."

But although the gambler may cite practical reasons for chasing, Rosenthal's research suggests more primal motivation. He says:

> Chasing is largely due to the patient's narcissistic entitlement, excessive competitiveness, or defenses against shame and guilt. Some gamblers believe that something is owed them, to make up for early deprivation and the 'unfairness' of the hand fate dealt them. Others speak of getting back "their" money, as if some valued part of the self had been abducted. This goes beyond issues of self-esteem; what is threatened is their very existence. For the more competitive gambler, losing is simply inconceivable.

One observation from Rosenthal hit me right between the eyes:

> The intense concentration involved in gambling, which blots out memories of everyday life, offers a kind of primitive avoidance, and a hiding out from the eyes of the world. At the same time, the social acceptance of the casino or race track denies one is disapproved of or an outcast.

Clearly there are no social clubs—such as the Knights at Hamilton High School—to reject you in the casino's happy neon universe.

Another expert on the compulsive gambler's psyche is Dr. Paul Good, a San Francisco psychologist whose practice initially focused on substance abuse cases but by 1990 dealt exclusively with gamblers. "Why is it," Good asked to illustrate a point, "that recreational gamblers and professional gamblers can just walk away from the tables?" The answer is no surprise: "They don't have their egos invested. They are not working out an emotional issue. They are not projecting an emotional issue onto the gambling. There is no imperative to stay." The compulsive gambler, on the other hand, "uses the gambling as an arena to play out his or her neuroses."

Through more than 175 clients, from various genders, ages, marital status, ethnicities, income, social status, and upbringing, Good has amassed a wealth of compulsive gambler "types" and rationales for engaging in an activity guaranteed to plunder their savings.

"You address the gambling behavior per se but you also have to examine and understand the neuroses," Good says. He is prepared to go wherever that neuroses leads—at times to Freud's conclusion in "Dostoyevsky and Patricide" that the gambler seeks to punish himself for his unconscious thoughts of wanting to kill his father. Gambling is a handy solution, since the gambler is guaranteed to suffer. Is such a theory, embraced by Bergler almost a half-century ago, outdated?

"For some gamblers," says Good, "it really fits." He continues, "One of the things we've observed in male gamblers is starting a gambling cycle soon after the death of the father. The death sets off the unconscious fantasy that the gambler has killed him, thereby stimulating the guilt that needs to be atoned for. The result is gambling and devastating losses. I have seen that in a few of my patients."

Although Good sees patients from all the typical gambling venues (casino, race track, sports betting, card clubs, etc) he was at the center of the "day-traders" craze in the mid-1990s, seeing a flood of patients who had sought to crack the Nasdaq. "A large majority of them wound up in serious debt," Good says. "Some as much as $200,000."

Day traders may have walked into the biggest scam since three-card monte or the Ponzi Scheme. In a *New Yorker* magazine article called "Striking It Rich" (January 14, 2002) John Cassidy writes:

The founder of All-Tech Investment Group once referred to day trading as "the best entertainment since television," but there was nothing entertaining about gullible investors losing their life savings. According to the Electronic Traders Association's own figures, the average day-trader bought or sold six million shares a year. Assuming that he paid two cents a share, which was common, he spent a hundred and twenty thousand dollars a year in commissions—more than many day-traders had in their accounts to begin with. Given these fees, the common perception that day trading was a relatively cheap business to operate was an illusion. Behind the marketing hype about personal empowerment, day trading was a business that any Wall Street old hand could appreciate: the customers risked their capital; the brokers made the profit.

The article included several poignant examples:

When the Massachusetts authorities investigated a day-trading firm in the state, they found that sixty-seven out of sixty-eight customers had lost money. Tales of disaster multiplied. A Chicago waiter with no trading experience blew a two-hundred-million-dollar inheritance. A Boston retiree went through two hundred and fifty thousand dollars of his wife's savings in a few hours. A California bank employee quit his job, borrowed forty thousand dollars on his credit cards to start trading and promptly lost the lot.

It's hard to know if day-trading's victims sought professional help; the alternatives (including "chasing") are all doomed to failure.

Although Good employs various methodologies for treating gambling addiction, he does not let society itself off the hook. "The existential element here is most profound," he says. "People are empty and unable in our society to have passion, to live in a meaningful and sensitive erotic kind of way."

Good says that gambling provides a "pseudo passion," even though it is described by many (including industry officials) as scintillating and exciting. "This desire to gamble seems to be a marvelous symbol of what's gone wrong in society," Good maintains. "We are suffering a loss of personal fulfillment. Winning money in a casino is really an attempt to alleviate the bankruptcy of the soul."

Research Sources

1) A Study of the Dopamine D2 Receptor Gene in Pathological Gambling. David E. Comings, Pharmocogenetics 6, 223-234, 1996.

2) Vincent Chiappinelli, addiction specialist, George Washington University Medical Center, Washington DC.

3) A Study of the Dopamine D2 Receptor Gene in Pathological Gambling. David E. Comings, Pharmocogenetics 6, 223-234, 1996.

4) The Molecular Genetics of Pathological Gambling, David E. Comings, MD.

5) Familial Influences on Gambling Behavior: An Analysis of 3359 Twin Pairs. Seth A. Eisen MD, Washington University School of Medicine, St. Louis MO. Research report, 1998.

6) The Genetics of Pathological Gambling. Seth Eisen, MD, Washington University School of Medicine, St. Louis MO, 1999.

Part 3

PROFILES

COMPULSIVE GAMBLERS COME IN ALL SHAPES, sizes, ethnicities, income, occupations, social status and ages. They usually fit into two categories: "action" and "escape relief." The former thrives on getting juiced up, watching the dice swirl on green felt, or squeezing an ace-ten on the blackjack table or urging the steel ball into the "00" hole on the roulette wheel. The escape relief gamblers, mostly women, find their thrill in slot machines, which provide total escape into a secret world. A seductive machine mesmerizes them by intermittently offering acceptance in the form of cash—metal coins that glitter and clink like costume jewelry.

Of course, there are subsets within the action and escape-relief gamblers. Following are real life cases of compulsive gamblers. As noted earlier, Gamblers Anonymous keeps no records and its critics place its success rate at a low percentage. However, as this profile section documents, many compulsive gamblers credit GA as being essential to their recovery. Pseudonyms and further masking of identities have been used with the exception of Patty and Mitzi Schlichter, both of whom have gone public with their stories.

Chapter 17

The Brit: Russell (age 52)

Psychiatrists and biologically oriented psychologists are now studying how gambling affects the brain. Some are researching the high state of arousal produced by gambling. Others are looking at brain wave patterns and chemical activity in the brain.

—Henry R. Lesieur, Ph.D.

RUSSELL'S THEORY OF THE GAMBLING BUG IS SIMPLE: There's a piece of the brain, he says, that pushes all logic away.

In Russell's case, it fits. How else to explain a man who spent his teenage years in London working in his father's bingo parlors, emptying the slot machines, and later moving up to croupier for dice and dealing blackjack? A man who studied accounting and knew every nuance about chance and probability and how the deck was stacked?

There's a charming lilt to Russell's British accent, in which all gamblers are "punters." But when Russell recounts his last few years in California, falling prey to the unregulated Indian casinos where the house edge verges on larceny, you wonder how he could have let $2 million slip through his fingers. So does he. It's insidious, he says. He was in denial.

Russell concedes that California's 1998 ballot Proposition 1A ("Indian Gambling Initiative") forced elimination of the $1 "rake" taken from each bet on a hand of blackjack. But for the four years prior to the initiative, a dollar was the "cost" to play a hand. If a gambler put down a five-dollar bet he'd be paying 20 percent interest on each hand. The slots, however, remain unregulated, as opposed to those in Nevada, where the state gaming commission insures a semblance of fairness.

Russell himself never had to worry about such steep interest, since his bets at blackjack were at the maximum, $300. Then he latched onto the dollar slot machines, going through $1,000-plus a day.

Russell's been "clean" just eight months, and the gambling scars are still raw. He recently filed for bankruptcy, closed his car dealership and has been in and out of the hospital for "stress-related problems." That's not hard to imagine, since Russell carries considerable bulk, usually camouflaged by untucked shirts draped over his middle. He walks at a decidedly acute angle, moving aggressively, making plans, charming his listeners with his appealing sure-footedness.

Russell's latest business scheme would have to be considered the "hair of the dog" variety. He wants to open a treatment center for compulsive gamblers—financed by the local gambling casinos. It's in the casinos' interest. Otherwise, he maintains, ten years down the road they'll be where the tobacco companies are now.

For a modicum of serenity, Russell merely needs to think back to 1992, when life was relatively sane and his business acumen had netted him the car dealership, an upscale air-conditioned Palm Springs home and a substantial bank account. There were newspaper articles then about "the possibility" of Indian casinos coming to the desert. If that happens, Russell joked, he'd better leave town. Eight years later he would observe that he was only half joking.

So far, Russell has adhered to his prime rule of living: He never related income to expenditure. Translation: The cash went out, whether it existed or not. (It could always be found.) Now he clings to that lifestyle by a thread.

It's easy to picture a slimmed-down Russell in his teens, honoring his father by obediently taking to gambling. Weekends he'd be at the family bingo parlors, where the punters observed London's odd rules about the slot machines: they could be played before bingo, during intermission, and after bingo, roughly two and one-half hours per night. The youth who emptied the slot machines got a blunt lesson: Every machine on every night was filled to the top with coins. After he moved up to blackjack dealer and craps croupier, Russell found the lesson etched even finer: The house never had a losing night.

School was hardly the place for a youngster of Russell's drive. Each school year produced a report card with the same comment: "He can do better." But Russell hated school. He had his own plan: a lifestyle for the rich, if not famous. And he lived it. After aborting an apprenticeship in accounting, Russell hit his mark in real estate.

"One of the Six Young High Risers in West End," trumpeted Real Estate News. Russell was 21, blessed with a talent for making money and a burning need to spend it. He lived in a posh flat, drove an Olds 442 with quadraphonic sound and had the first car phone. But as fast as he was making it he was losing it.

Russell's casinos of choice in London were Charlie Chester's and the new plush Playboy Club. Dice and blackjack were Russell's favorites; heady action was the rule at Charlie Chesters, a modest-sized, family-owned, smoke-filled casino done up in shiny black and white walls with mirrors throughout. The British pounds flew feverishly, transformed into chips and wagered amid a clubby atmosphere. In fact, you had to join Charlie Chester's before you were permitted entry; rule number 4 in a book of rules called *Charlie Chester Casino Club* stated that "Ladies and gentlemen of good social position over the age of eighteen years are eligible for membership of the Club." They even had a modest dress code.

Here Russell came night after night, despite his earlier training in the folly of nonstop gambling action. He managed to lose even more than was coming in. His credit line was easily stretched since he did business with the same bank as his father. In those days you could overdraft, so he'd cash huge checks at the Playboy Club until the bank got wise.

The bank cut off Russell's credit—they wanted what he owed. It took him two long years to get even with the bank. Did he have a gambling "problem?"

He didn't know about Gamblers Anonymous or that he was sick. But Russell knew he wanted to get away from gambling.

The very day he got even with the bank, his roommate announced he was going to the States. Russell made a snap decision to go "for a month" and purchased a round-trip ticket. He was 25, free of debt, and didn't want to gamble anymore. Only half the plane ticket was put to use.

For his first twenty years in the United States Russell gorged on the American Dream. He landed first in southern California, where he took up residence on a friend's couch. After two weeks he realized he needed a car. So he went to a dealership in Culver City and got both car and job. His London salesmanship skills served him well; he flourished. Next he got into the clothing business in Venice, California.

Along the way Russell met and married Susan. Did he talk about his gambling? He told her nothing about it, Russell says with a tinge of sadness. He was not aware that he had a problem. But he'd learn the truth—eventually.

For the next sixteen years Russell's gambling was confined to two annual flings in Las Vegas or Reno. He might blow $1,000, but with his income that was nothing serious. If the casinos were closer, Russell said at the time, it would have been a problem.

That statement, of course, was prescient. After his Venice Beach clothing store was demolished to make room for a mall, Russell had an offer to open a store in Palm Springs. Again, he flourished; to the retail clothes store he added a car dealership. Life was good. For a while.

Russell would be hard pressed to identify California's Mission Indians, but they were tied to his future. The U.S. Supreme Court in 1987 issued its *California v. Cabazon Band of Mission Indians* decision, in essence saying the states had no right to regulate gambling on Native American reservations. Congress quickly passed the Indian Gaming Regulatory Act (1988), an attempt at regulating the casinos and requiring that gambling revenues promote "economic development and welfare" of tribes.

But what it meant for Palm Springs residents was a casino on Palm Canyon Drive, the town's main street, and two more just outside of town. Russell's life veered out of control. The part of his brain that "pushes all logic away" took over. With his family life in tatters, Russell simply headed to Vegas for bigger play. And even though he hit the gambler's supreme payoff—something the odds say you'd wait a thousand years for—that did not assuage the pain of addiction. It happened at the Tropicana Hotel, around noontime.

Russell had cashed in a C note ($100) and got four quarters ($25 chips). He was playing Baccarat, the classy game of European origin where the dealers wear tuxedoes and champagne replaces beer. The high stakes game is also incredibly rapid; there are no decisions, just the "player" or the "bank" trying to get closest to a total of 9 in two (a "natural") or three cards. You can bet on the bank or the player, the latter Russell's choice. The "shoe" holds eight decks, and when Russell sat down with his puny $100 it was as if the Gods of Gambling had struck him with a bolt of magic. The eight decks contained an incredible run of 27 straight wins for the player.

When it played out, Russell had run his $100 into $78,000! The house big shots were grateful that Russell hadn't hit that stretch of luck a few hours later, when the big players drop in. It would have broken the hotel. But Russell would later say he outsmarted himself. The gambler's dream would be drained of meaning. He cashed in for $50,000 and played out the rest. Which he lost quickly. Russell thought he was using logic. He was smart. He quit. Walked out. The worst part of having a stake of $50K, Russell admits, was knowing it was there. He fed off it. He could think of little else. It was soon depleted.

But the bad luck run provided something positive—a psychic jolt that forced Russell to assess his pattern. He could go on "tilt" (gamble insanely) or seek help. It did not require a coin flip. The local GA chapter welcomed its newest member. Russell found his freedom in sharing his woeful tales of addiction. In fact, it was at a GA meeting that Russell came to a profoundly simple realization, which he scribbled on a piece of paper: "YCW."

"You can't win," he says stoically. The big score doesn't settle anything. You're addicted to the thrill, Russell reasons. It's simple. He recites his new mantra: *You Can't Win!*

Postscript: I caught up with Russell a few years down the road. He had managed to keep his home and was about to open another car dealership. Debts had been paid. A lesson had been learned despite the brain's trick of often working against the addict.

Chapter 18

The Caretaker: Patty (age 40)

The tremendous concentration and focus in gambling blots out aware-
ness of outside problems, a kind of temporary amnesia, as the individual
gets lost in the artificial world of play.

—Dr. Richard Rosenthal

PATTY'S SAGA BEGAN (AND NEARLY ENDED) when she left her family a voice mail message that crackled with resolve:

"The papers are in the truck. I'm useless as a mother. You're better off without me."

Patty was not bluffing. She had a gun. She had pills. And there was a street full of traffic she could dart into. In fact, she had staggered out of the Palm Springs bar and was headed for her favorite gambling haunt. She was going to shoot herself, right in front of the casino. Patty was intercepted by a lanky teenager who grabbed her by the shoulders and shoved her against the wall. "You've got responsibilities," Patty's assailant told her. "And I'm one of them." Shaken, Patty stared into the eyes of David, her 16-year-old son.

Patty's husband, A.J., and David had picked the bar near the casino to search for Patty after the desperate phone message—even though Patty had left home that night with $100 cash and a promise "to go grocery shopping." Patty knew that was her last night of gambling. She had written a string of bad checks, had borrowed and stolen from every available source. She had blown the $100 food money in no time. She was thousands of dollars in debt.

What she didn't know is that she would crawl back from the brink. That six months later she would rejoin the living and that she would unabashedly tell all—to the news media, to other gambling addicts—and even appear on a TV talk show along with A.J.

I've nothing to be ashamed of, Patty says now. She was emotionally addicted—an escape-relief gambler. Translation: Patty would shove mountains of coins into the slot machines for hours on end. When the money ran out she needed a fix—cash was all that mattered. Before her two-year skid into addiction ended, Patty was pilfering money from her son's sock drawer. Always, she points out, with the intent of replacing it—even adding a little extra. She was sure she was going to win. Patty says her life in the throes of addiction was "one big lie." And the biggest lie was that the solution to her problems lay in winning.

A year before our interviews, Patty was sitting on the dais of a Seattle TV talk show along with husband A.J. Patty's questioners in the studio audience were incredulous. What could Patty the "escape-relief" gambler possibly want to escape from?

It was a fair question, since Patty comes across as upbeat, articulate, maternal, rational, sensitive. "I felt," Patty said with eyes moist, "that someone else had taken over my body." She described "slot machines calling me back. They grabbed hold of me like a monster. It's like you can't breathe. You're constantly thinking about the machines." She shakes her head now in disbelief, red hair brushing her shoulders.

Patty's first step toward gambling addiction was innocent enough. "My mother-in-law asked me to accompany her to a bingo game. She said it would be fun. So I went." Patty had the misfortune to win $600. Later that night she hit big time, squeezing $4,000 out of the local casino's slot machines. "It was a real rush," she recalls. "I thought that this was the solution to my money problems."

Although the wins led Patty to her descent into gambling addiction, the origins began decades earlier.

Her childhood bubble of innocence burst at age five. "I had this kidney problem," Patty recalls, suffused with shame at the memory. "I was a . . . wetter." Predictably, the other children teased without mercy. "They were cruel. I felt inadequate. That I could never do anything on my own."

Patty's way of coping was to become the perfect little child. "So I lost me. By being there for everyone else, I lost my identity. I reached out for everyone else." Between the imperfect kidney and her own attempt to be perfect, Patty was a conflicted and unhappy child. She found her purpose in "fixing" others—and winning their approval. While her four older siblings moved on with their lives, Patty dropped out of high school and soon drifted into drugs and alcohol. "But I never went over the line," she says in her own defense. "I never got too drunk or too stoned."

Then at age 18 Patty visited Reno. It was her first brush with a reliable companion—the nickel slot machines. "I wasn't into gambling then," she continues. "But when I look back at it now I see that I had all the characteristics of the compulsive gambler. I remember just loving it." What she loved most was being able to "zone out." "I could shut down my brain. I didn't have to think about how I looked. Was I too fat? Was I pretty? I always worried about what other people thought of me. Worried about what to say to people. But with the slot machines I didn't have to." Patty recalls that on subsequent trips to casinos others would joke about lodgings. "Why bother getting a room for her?" they would say. "She's always at the slot machines." Recalls Patty: "I just loved the fact that I didn't have to converse. I was free to think what I wanted, when I wanted."

Patty hooked up with a crowd that shared her gambling rush. "I started dating this guy who loved to gamble," she recalls. "We'd close the bar at 2 a.m. and drive to Laughlin (a tiny Nevada gambling spot), gamble four or five hours and be back by noon." Patty would park herself in front of her game of choice, the slot machine. "I didn't have the guts to try craps or blackjack," she confesses. "I felt intimidated. Afraid to screw up in front of people."

Patty's relationship with the slot machines at this period was strictly platonic. "When it was time to stop we stopped." She was now 29 with two young children, two marriages gone sour, struggling financially as a waitress. Her gambling trips became more frequent. Patty got hired as a bartender, where she met a number of intense men. She started dating one who had the gambling habit—bad. "He'd be at Indio for the satellite wagering or the racetrack or Reno." When Tom won he was generous; when he lost he was best avoided. "He started running up big gambling debts," Patty says. "He was talking on the phone to bookies all the time. I finally realized that this guy's bad news."

Did she not see Tom's gambling antics as a cautionary tale?

"No," Patty says firmly. "That was *his* problem."

But Patty ceased dating for a long time.

Then one night she stopped at a local bar after work and met A.J. "It started as a deep friendship," she says. "We went out that night," Patty says with great relief. "And from then on I dated no one else." In her marriage sweepstakes, third time proved the charm. Fortunately for Patty's "fix them" self, A.J. wasn't perfect. He drank. "It wasn't constant. It was from the time he entered the bar until the time they threw him out. Another 'fix-it' case. Plus he had a violent side—but never against me. He punched his windshield out."

Patty recalls A.J.'s last drinking bout. "He got us both drunk once and got us arrested. That was it. A.J. quit drinking. He was fixed." By Patty's own reckoning, her "fix-it" self was no longer in need. "What does Patty do?" she asks herself. "Patty breaks herself and thinks that she doesn't belong here." It was the same year that Indian casinos came to town. The mix was volatile; it was 1994.

From all appearances, Patty's life with A.J., though not perfect, was stable. But things quickly went downhill. "I was devastated in less than two years," she says. The big question was *why*? "I was used to the turmoil.

Without it I had to focus on me." Since it was unbearable to focus on her unresolved conflicts, she opted for escape. Soon the slots would be calling her name. Asked to cite the moment she stepped over the line, breaking her own ethical/moral code with the family's money, Patty becomes reflective. "It's hard to say when you cross that line. Because if you did you'd catch yourself."

With substance abuse Patty saw the line clearly and would bounce back to acceptable behavior. "I didn't do drugs or alcohol to destroy myself, I did it to escape." Gambling was different. "Gambling sneaks up on you. I didn't see the line. The first time I realized it was a problem was when I bounced a check. I thought I better do something to take care of this." Patty deliberately wrote no checks in the casinos so A.J. wouldn't suspect the degree of her addiction. "But then," Patty says, "I realized that I could not go two days without visiting the casino. I'm not stupid. I knew this was a problem but I thought I could take care of it."

As Patty's gambling increased so did tensions with her teenage daughter. "I was out of giving," Patty says. "I had no more left. That's probably when I realized I had crossed the line." Patty got in deeper and deeper. "With drugs and alcohol as soon as it looked like I was going to hurt someone, I'd stop. But this was different." Patty pauses, revealing a jolting insight: "I was taking everyone down with me. I was hurting them like I'd been hurt all my life." Patty borrowed from everyone available—even her social security-dependent parents. She borrowed from her mother in law, her friends, her co-workers. Patty miraculously kept her family off her trail by lying about where she'd been.

"I should have been a scholar," she says with gallows humor, "for all the time I said I'd been at the library." Once she did stop at the library to grab a book and bolster her story. "Oh," A.J. asked her. "Are you interested in accounting?" Patty grabbed that book simply because it was in the A's, and handy. "I would leave the casino, broke and emotionally wrenched, and rehearse in my mind the excuses I'd use. It was like writing a play. I'd imagine what I'd say and what A.J. would say." Eventually Patty felt trapped. "I realized that I didn't love going to the casinos, it was that I *needed* to go. I couldn't face life. I had no reason. And I didn't care anymore."

After the aborted suicide attempt outside the bar when she was accosted by her son David, Patty staggered toward the car and agreed to return home. A.J. told her the marriage was basically over unless she sought help for her addiction.

He offered her the guest room, but that night she slept on the couch. "I spent the night shaking," Patty recalls during our interview, day 981 of being "clean." She and A.J. had reconciled once she agreed that her gambling days were behind her and that together they would face their creditors. Patty's bounced checks were now her responsibility. "You go face those people," A.J. had told her. And she did. She also had a huge hospital bill (not gambling-related) but arranged to pay it back in installments, admitting that she had a gambling problem. A.J. doled out to his wife only the money that she needed.

"At first it was humiliating," Patty admits. "Then it was comforting. Then he said, 'I trust you.' But," she wondered, "do I trust myself?" Patty had the sudden revelation that "it's okay for me to have a problem. It's okay for someone to help me. I was like a newborn child."

Soon adult Patty became a stickler with the checkbook. Bills were paid on time. "I discovered that saving was good." She also discovered a welcome truth about herself one bright afternoon when she was on the way to the bank with $900 cash and made a wrong turn. "I realized I was near the casino," she says. "But there wasn't even a question of going in."

As she nears 1,000 days of gambling sobriety, Patty says that "most of them have been glorious. With their ups and downs, of course. Life is life. "Before I ran from everything. Now I don't run from anything."

Chapter 19

The Judge: Jake (age 50)

Through the free, independent self-regulation of action gamblers confirm their existence. They prove to themselves over and over again that they are alive by speeding up their heart rate and increasing their muscle tension and by becoming emotionally aroused either positively—with hope, for example—or negatively—perhaps with anxiety.

—Igor Kusyszn

JAKE HAD AN AMUSING SENSE OF PROPORTION. "If I had all the money in the world," he said, "I would have to move to a different world." Jake's not your typical compulsive gambler—or person. He turned down interview requests from *60 Minutes* and *20-20* TV magazine shows. "I didn't want to put my family through any more publicity." We spoke several times by phone, Jake eager to tell his story provided his identify was masked.

Jake was a legend—from the glitzy Las Vegas gambling tables to the staid municipal court where he held forth in black robes with upright bearing. How he managed this double life seems the stuff of fiction. But it was real.

Jake once placed second in a Las Vegas blackjack tournament, pocketing $96,000. Queried back home about his big time gambling lifestyle, Jake saw no conflict. "It's OK to gamble in Las Vegas," he said. "It's legal there." The Mirage Hotel had banned Jake after a 13-month win streak. Jake boasted a towering one-day win at the MGM Grand Hotel of a million dollars. He even tipped the dealer $60,000. Hours later he'd be on the bench, admonishing attorneys, advising witnesses and deciding fates of defendants. It was a frenetic life under firm control.

But where were the clues that Jake would switch from skilled player to desperate addict? What would cause him to jettison his edge (he was a skilled card-counter) and hover on the rim of ruin? Surely not his mid-West upbringing, where family values such as "honesty, loyalty and hard work" were drummed into Jake and his two younger siblings. He oozes praise for both parents.

"My father was a brilliant guy," Jake says, "even though he did not see himself that way. He quit school because the family needed the income. He won a Bronze Star in World War II. He did drink, though. A functioning alcoholic." Jake's mother was reared in poverty. "She placed a big value on education." Jake was the first in the family to attend college. His mother never tired of starting conversations with: "Have I told you about my son the judge?" Jake had reached that pinnacle at age 27—the youngest municipal court judge in the state.

But Jake was also quirky. A microbiology major in college, he rejected medical school because "the application forms were too long." He opted for an accelerated law school program. But after leaping every law school hurdle and finishing in a record 23 months, Jake hit a brick wall: a regulation was changed and he was denied his degree. What did the precocious legal mind do? He sued. Jake took on the state's highest court and won. After a brief stint as a public defender, he got an appointment to the bench. There he gestated for a solid decade: the sober, deliberating judge, the involved family man, the pillar of the community. He was a little league dad, a physical fitness nut, a techno guru. Jake was characterized by a colleague as having "a brilliant mind, an engaging personality." He joined the elite country club but was a soft touch for charitable causes.

His was a life to inspire envy. But Jake wasn't satisfied. His brilliant mind sought frenzy. And it came in one flavor. Jake had metamorphosed into the classic action gambler. He had abandoned his card counting scheme, which required full concentration, in favor of pure chance—which sent his adrenalin into mach speed.

When he lost, Jake says, "I had this unrelenting pain. I had to get back into action as fast as I could." And when he wasn't "in action"? "I would drift into a very deep depression." He admitted to spasms of "attention deficit disorder," a common thread among pathological gamblers. To stave off the depression— and light the frenzy—Jake indulged his gambling passion. But not even the judge was prepared for the consequences. (Asked some time later if he had ever lied to his wife about his gambling habit, Jake laughs: "The times I told the truth were rare. I always lied. My life was one big lie.")

The Vegas trips became more frequent. The string of big wins was behind him. People in town talked; they wondered. Jake was sliding down the slope of addiction. An enormous mountain of debt threatened to bury him—along with his high-achiever lifestyle. He took risks. He stopped being careful. He grabbed any cash within reach—no matter whose. As soon as the local press got a whiff of "public wrongdoing by a judge," he was ripe for plucking. The headlines, stories, analyses and editorials whipped up local indignation. "Authorities Raid Court After Top Judge Quits/Records Seized in Wake" screamed one headline early in the onslaught. Jake had tried to resign for "health reasons." But no one bought that, and his life turned into a nightmare. He had embezzled, he had taken kickbacks, he had laundered money, he had scammed—all to keep checks flying to cover losses. The community reacted with moral outrage. A judge cheating? Committing crimes?

Months of headlines culminated in the one that pitched Jake into the world of perps: JUDGE DRAWS 8-YEAR SENTENCE.

For his "own protection," Jake was sentenced to a prison out of state. He spent one year in medium-security, housed with 15 others—11 serving time for murder. "The former judge has learned to watch his back, sleep lightly and wake up every morning knowing that today is going to be nearly identical to the past 1,100 days," a newspaper article said. Then they quoted Jake: "I'm not sure we're doing anybody a great favor in giving them a life sentence over the death penalty . . . I'd have to think twice if I were in that position."

The judge turned perp was "hot copy." More than 150 articles poured out of the local newspaper, cataloging every crime, every plea bargain, every person Jake had victimized.

Next came the jail cell interviews. "I didn't believe that the rules did or should apply to me," he said of his life before prison. "In prison, you don't have that luxury. At any time, anyone can go through your personal property. There are no guarantees, and there is no right of privacy."

In another interview Jake was more succinct: "I've got it," he said. "I understand, I really do. And the only thing that's going to be served by keeping me in here is more punishment for my family and loved ones." From prison, Jake talked often about his children: "I've become my son's greatest fear," Jake revealed. "He worries that the newspapers won't stop printing bad things about me." He could turn ironic: "Years ago," he said, "I was worried my children were going to grow up too privileged, that they wouldn't have the proper perspective on life, and I was thinking of what I needed to teach them about the value of money. Well, I certainly solved that one."

People wondered if Jake was still scamming—this time for benefit of the Parole Board. The board rejected his appeal the first time around. But when he neared the halfway point in his eight-year sentence, they softened. Jake finally saw the headline that ended his agony: Ex-Judge Granted Parole/Board Bets He Will Pay Restitution.

The TV news magazines clamored for Jake's story. He declined. "No more publicity for my family," he said. "They've been through enough." He agreed to be interviewed for this book (with identifying details changed) for the simplest of reasons: to help others escape—or avoid—the painful grip of addiction.

Although Jake sees futility in discovering the "Why" of his own addiction, he acknowledges his early attraction to gambling. He played penny-ante gin rummy with his mother. Then at age 13 he discovered "a native ability with poker." From there, Jake says, "it was off to the races."

He gambled all the way through high school. One poker game stands out in stark relief—a game that should have been a clue.

"I had just graduated high school. Bought this car for $100. Got into the game with $95. Ran it up to $390. Wanted to get the next ten dollars. Then quit—at $400. A winner! But I chased the ten down to nothing. Lost everything. Everything! Driving home I was pounding the steering wheel: 'How could you be so stupid?'"

Jake has a sequel: "Fast forward 25 years. Coming over the bridge. Had been to Vegas. Had to get back to the bank and reload before she (my wife) got there: I'm $800,000 in the hole. Wanted to win a million. I was $10,000 away! Chased the $10,000 down to nothing. Lost everything! Driving away, hitting steering wheel: 'How could you be so stupid?' The only difference was I was driving a $95,000 car."

With perfect hindsight, Jake concludes: "It's never about the money. If I had won all the money in the world, I would have had to move to a different world."

Jake has more than his share of regret: "I could have retired last July with a six-figure income," he says. "But I made some bad choices." Jake has no illusions: "I had every opportunity in the world," he says. "And I wasted them all." If there's any redemption in Jake's story, it's the satisfaction he derives in counseling today's problem gamblers.

"I don't counsel," Jake corrects. "I chat. I tell them it's not as bad as they think."

And if the hooked gambler says he wants to quit but doesn't know if he can?

"I tell him not to go there. Don't speak in absolutes. Let's break this thing in small parts. Let's have lunch. Can you not gamble for one hour? Two hours? Once you get a couple of hours in, you go for a day. Then two days. Keep your eye on the ball. Then I suggest they attend a GA meeting. It's a process."

The goal, of course is to get some distance between the "now" and that last bet. Jake—like many recovering gamblers—can pinpoint the date. "Seven years ago—pre-prison," he says. "I lost $10,000 on a hand of blackjack. I busted with a queen."

Jake credits Gamblers Anonymous (a condition of his early prison release) for his recovery. "If I had just gone to prison," he says. "I would have come out the same arrogant prick. I could not have done it without GA. It was talking with other gamblers. I need that social structure of support."

As if Jake needed any testimonials, he got one from the head of the state's gambling council: "The former arrogant, egotistical, narcissistic and controlling Jake has been replaced. The new Jake demonstrates remorse for his actions. He no longer needs to be the center of attention."

Still, many would write Jake off as a sociopath—a person caught up in his own world without a thought for the welfare of anyone else. It would take perhaps another compulsive gambler—someone who has tasted the sweet flame of addiction—to accept Jake's own take on himself.

"I'm not a bad guy," Jake says. "I'm a good guy who did bad things."

Chapter 20

The System Player:
Josh (age 52)

If all my bets were safe there just wouldn't be any juice.
—Axel in *The Gambler* by James Toback

JOSH IS ONE OF THOSE GAMBLERS WHO HAS MORE TO WORRY ABOUT than the house edge. He got caught up in a "system" for sale. Josh soon learned that this is worse than the house edge. Winning information is always "guaranteed," meaning if it's bad you get some more. Josh is clearly too smart to fall for such snake oil, but he did.

Gamblers love systems. The house loves them even more—especially a craps system, where there is no variation. There are six ways to make a seven and one way to make a 2 ("snake eyes") or 12 ("boxcars"). And that's that.

Card counters and handicappers can often make a case for an "edge." But a dice system? Josh claims he found one. "I saw this ad in the newspaper," he told me. "'Winning Craps System! Learn Professionally!' I sent them $400. Got all the books, charts, videos. A ton of stuff. Studied the system for six months. It was very complicated. But I mastered it." Was this the gambler's Holy Grail? Josh would find out.

He headed for Nevada's green felt testing ground. Josh stuck with the system for one month. "I won about $11,000," he says. "But I was miser-able. It did not allow me to be 'in action'." Josh "tweaked" the rules. Where the system said "stop and wait until the next day" he'd plunge in. "The dice didn't know it wasn't a new day," he reasoned. Result: his financial resources were drained.

It's a familiar ring. Most systems produce slowly; problem gamblers often describe playing them "like working." Dull, predictable bets provide no "juice." You become studious, bored.

Josh traded what seemed like a sure thing for the pumped up thrill of risk. He shared another of the gambler's special traits: superstition. His football betting saga sounds like something from Ripley's *Believe It or Not!* "I knew there was no logic to it," he says, "but every time my girlfriend's mother phoned the house my team would blow the lead." Things got so predictable he would forbid her to call on game day. But she foiled his plan, as the Baltimore Colts were three touchdowns ahead "one gorgeous Sunday when everything was going right." He'd hit the first three games of the parlay. Once the Colts held up their end Josh would realize a major payday—without leaving the house. But when Josh heard Gail say "Hi, Mom," he went into a rage. Sure enough, his team crumbled.

Josh is an intelligent man who studied business and marketing at a prestigious university. He knew his "superstitious behavior" was absurd. He also recognized his addictive behavior: "As long as I was in action, I felt comfort. I kept throwing bets out there. And it got worse. I maxed out my credit cards, one after another." Deeper debt meant more action was needed "to dig my way out." Josh called in his bets like a man begging for oxygen; there were just enough "solid blips" (win bets) on the radar screen to keep him alive. But if Josh stopped to peer through the haze of addiction he could see the inevitable—stupefying losses that would end the game. He preferred the haze.

Looking back at his initial gambling experiences, Josh saw "intriguing possibilities."

He was ten. "The typical card games," Josh says. "Playing blackjack for pennies. Pitching nickels and dimes." A few years later a camping trip ended up in a blackjack game, with Josh taking the deal. "We played for dollars and quarters. I got real intrigued, winning $12 on one trip. All the way back home, a six-hour drive, I was counting my money. I had enough for a new skateboard."

Josh had three older siblings in a family steeped in alcoholism—two brothers and his mother were addicted—yet the youngest son managed to function in a dysfunctional setting. The family's restaurant supply business provided for basic needs. And Josh attended first-rate Catholic schools where discipline and regard for learning were paramount. So it was not out of financial necessity that Josh felt compelled to score after-school jobs. During high school he was a busboy and a dishwasher. Then he hit the big time when he landed a ballboy job with the local NFL team.

Josh recalls that era with a mix of nostalgia and dread. "This one player was heading to the county fair where they had horse racing and said he had 'inside information' on one race. All the players gave him money to bet for them. I gave him some, too." Josh was swept away when the player returned and handed him $40. "Hey," Josh recalled thinking, "this is so easy. This is great." When the local racetrack opened for the season, Josh became the bet-taker for the players. "I made these trips to the track, twice a week, for two years." But Josh also learned something unpleasant about himself. "I got sneaky." Translation: "For certain people, I would not bet their horse. I'd just keep the money. If they won, I'd tell them I wasn't able to make the bet." One player hit the daily double (first two races) for $140. Josh simply said "I didn't get to the track on time. I basically bullshitted the guy." Was Josh believed? "I'm not sure."

Still a teenager, Josh had landed a job as a waiter. The restaurant owner took the whole crew to Harrah's beautiful lakeside casino hotel. "I didn't gamble," Josh recalled. "But I heard all the bells and whistles in the casino."

Not many years later Josh would frequent that same casino. A robust, athletic young man, Josh was an avid skier. "Pretty soon I did less and less skiing and more gambling. I couldn't wait to get off the slopes and into the casino." The ride home was predictable: "I was depressed and broke." When his current job provided insufficient gambling funds, Josh would slip "a ten or a twenty" from his father's drawer. He even confronted his addiction, telling his father, "I think I have a gambling problem." His father dismissed the idea. "He had his head in the sand," Josh says in hindsight. Working in the family business, Josh found pilfering an easy matter. More losses, more pilfering.

Josh's gambling habit increased. This time he turned to a type of system that always spells doom—buying information from "experts" on sports wagering. Josh shelled out several hundred dollars. These picks are always "guaranteed"; if your team should lose, they give you a free pick. That should have been enough of a clue for someone of Josh's intelligence to smell scam. "They also nicked you for $50 per phone call," Josh adds, "and I'd sometimes make the call at a customer's phone, dialing the 900 number, for which the customer would pay." Josh concedes he wasn't "very happy" with himself about stiffing his father's clients.

Logic always suggests that touts who sell information—whether on horses or sport events—would do better to bet their picks rather than sell them. Josh religiously played the purchased "information," and got further in debt. Years later he spotted his "source" on an NBC *Dateline* TV exposé. "These guys all worked out of one office in Palm Springs," Josh says with unsubtle amusement. "I thought he was up in Oregon. That's where I placed the calls." The more "valuable" the information, the bigger the price. "And," Josh explained slightly incredulously, "at one point the *Dateline* undercover cameras showed how the 'pro handicapper' figured out the winner—he flipped a coin!" Josh recalls when he quit the touts and their bogus info that it wasn't easy to be rid of them. "They'd keep phoning me. Even after I moved a few times. They'd find me somehow and try to sell me tips. Offering me special deals." Josh was even solicited from casinos in the Caribbean; he was a marked man, and people wanted his business.

How Josh extricated himself from debt, addiction and pain is a testament to one man's determination. "I saw all these friends of mine buying houses and cars and I realized I had nothing. I had the same education they had. I had a good job. All my money went to gambling." Josh took a cold look at his own family history. "I realized that addiction or compulsion are hereditary," he says. His family members proved that.

But recognizing one's addiction and cracking the gambling habit are vastly different. It took a divorce and colossal losses to stoke Josh's desire for a gambling-free life. He'd blown "a couple hundred thousand in two years" but realized finally, "I could not take the pain anymore." The pain was induced by "all nighters" in Reno. "Vegas hotels comped me for everything—meals, rooms." Josh had ascended to the status of high roller; the clubs get very generous with high rollers, wanting desperately to take their action. Weekdays Josh could be found in Nevada; weekends he was home for sports wagering, truly a 24/7 habit. But the pain of loss—and dishonest methods of securing cash—became overwhelming. An emotional wreck, Josh amazingly crawled out from under his debilitating habit.

A testament to his sincerity, Josh recently marked five years since his last bet—a $1,200 wager on an NFL team that blew the point spread on a last-second field goal.

Josh gives high praise to his weekly Gamblers Anonymous meetings. But abstinence is not always easy. "It's still grinding it out. A day at a time." The gambling habit was hard to eradicate. It had worked its way into Josh's bloodstream. "It was a natural part of my life. I loved it. Or thought I did."

In his half-decade at GA meetings, Josh has gained even more insight on his addiction. "You think it's about the money," he says. "New people come into the program and they talk about the money they're losing. But it's never about the money. It's simply about being in action. It's about withdrawing from the world—the world of personal responsibility."

Chapter 21

The Loser: Arnie (age 52)

Many gamblers think they have been singled out by fate as a target for cruel jokes. They feel that they alone in all the universe are being tortured, experimented upon by some unknown force.

—Mike Caro

ARNIE HAD HIS OWN THEORY OF ECONOMICS.

He had racked up $90,000 in credit card debt, mortgaged his home, sold his car and somehow found the wisdom to contact an attorney. "She told me to file for bankruptcy and stop making all payments."

Arnie took it as a sign. "Gee," he says looking back, "now I'd have more money to gamble with." He took early retirement and a bundle of severance pay. "Now I had no bills to pay and more gambling money." He seemed to be living out the Horatio Alger story in reverse. A foreclosure on his house was not the voice of doom but simply a sign to move into a smaller place and take the equity cash from the house, and then he'd have "more money to gamble with."

It was hard to know when Arnie would finally recognize the "stop gambling" alert. He seemed to have a perverse take on his inability to pocket some winnings. Whereas most compulsive gamblers recall at least one monster win, Arnie seemed to take pride in the opposite. "See that ashtray," he'd say to house guests. "That ashtray cost me $1600. See that glass mug? That cost me $2300." The trinkets, of course, were "free" souvenirs from the casinos. How did Arnie explain his propensity for financial risk with no chance of coming out on top? He says it was the "gambling gene."

Actually his theory is broader than that; Arnie believes that he and his siblings were stuck with "the magic gene" that resulted in a variety of compulsive behavior, most notably alcoholism. "My half-brother had none of this obsessive stuff," Arnie says. "Us other kids—a brother and sister—did." His father was an alcoholic. For Arnie, gambling would be his undoing, but booze certainly helped grease the skid.

A stop at the local pub used to mean a man might just stagger home to an irate wife. But Arnie's Washington state pub also had "jugs," betting pull tabs where you could win up to $500, depending on the amount risked. Arnie would return both inebriated and broke.

Gambling was a lifestyle choice for Arnie that was first associated with family fun. He grew up in a family anchored by a mother who had lived through the dregs of the Depression. "She had scraped for every nickel," Arnie says. "We didn't have all the things other kids had, but we got by. We did a lot of outdoors stuff. We'd go deer hunting in Nevada and always stop for breakfast in Reno. No matter which restaurant we stopped in, there were slot machines. Our parents would let each kid pick out a slot machine and they'd give us $5 that they would play for us." Each child was given the chance of stopping when they were ahead or playing the money back. "I never wanted to stop," Arnie says. "I'd have them keep playing until every coin was gone."

Arnie's early gambling inclinations were easily satisfied. "As far back as elementary school I remember pitching pennies against the wall," he says. In junior high school it was flipping coins and pitching for quarters and sometimes dollars. Later, in high school, it was poker games, bowling "pot" games and shooting pool. When queried about academics, Arnie recalls school mainly "as a time of confusion." He strayed from college prep courses and chose instead furniture repair, metal shop, and wood shop.

Most compulsive gamblers recalling adolescence focus on big wins and the competition. Not Arnie: "I almost always lost," he says. "When I'd go into the pool hall the other guys would hold up their pool sticks like they were fishing poles and point at me—the fish." [Fish, in gambling parlance, means sucker.] Arnie could not get his money out fast enough. "It always wound up in their pockets."

He recalls one memorable teenage gambling trip to Reno. "A bunch of us took the bus," he says. He may have set a record even for Arnie: "I lost all my money at the bus station slot machines. I never even got to the casino."

Even Arnie concedes that marriage to a woman with three children "was a signal to slow down my gambling." They met at a local pub. "I liked her smile," Arnie says. "She thought I was a drug dealer." It was an honest mistake, since in those days—the mid-1980s—Arnie had long scraggly hair and a beard.

At 25 Arnie was a heavy mobile equipment mechanic at the Mare Island Ship Yard. He appeared to be Mr. Family Man. But everything in his life was subordinated to gambling. "This disease that I had inherited had this hold on me," he says. "I knew that it would not be long before I was back to my old ways."

The action was just a phone call away. "I'd bet with the bookie on weekend football games—college games on Saturday, the pros on Sunday. Then I'd bet three hundred to five hundred dollars on Monday Night Football to get even with what I lost on the weekend." What Arnie recalls for sure is that "I never had a winning season."

In the midst of this sea of financial red ink, Arnie stooped to what's known as a "betting service." For a fee, a gambling "expert" will give you scientifically handicapped "picks." Just a tad of logic would convince a gambler that if the betting service was an ace handicapper he wouldn't waste time selling his picks; he'd bet on them himself. The "picks" are always guaranteed; if the team (or horse) loses, you get a replacement pick. What you lose on the original pick is your problem.

"Pretty soon I was paying so much for the service that I didn't have money left to make my bets," Arnie recalls. "So I stopped the betting service." But the betting service honcho had all the integrity of a telemarketer. "They kept calling me back to buy more picks," Arnie says, somewhat amused. "I told them I didn't have a bookie anymore. Anything to get them off my back." But they suggested that Arnie go to a barber shop, a surefire place to find a bookie.

The message finally flashed in Arnie's brain when he had bet $1,000 each with two different bookies. "I realized," he says, "that if my team lost I couldn't pay off without selling something. That's when I knew I had a gambling problem."

But "knowing" and "stopping" are vastly different. Instead of stopping, Arnie devised creative tactics to hide his true income from his family. "My wife had started watching my pay stubs and having me account for every dime." So he took out a deposit at his credit union and had his paycheck routed there before it was sent home. "Every time I got a raise I'd have it show up on my pay stub as 'other allotments.' I'd tell my wife that money was going for insurance. It was the first time I'd deceived someone about my gambling."

Arnie's rationale for such deception is a variation on the compulsive gambler's credo—"I'm the victim." "She was always spending money on junk for the kids," Arnie said. "So I decided that I needed more money to gamble with. That was my way of having entertainment." Arnie's periodic gambling trips to Reno now included a hidden stake of $500 or $600. And he played everything: dice, roulette, poker, keno, blackjack and, what he calls his "big downfall"—slot machines. "I went from nickel and dime machines to quarters and dollars. Then I discovered the $5 machines. I'd hit some jackpots for $1500 or $2500 but they'd sure eat up the winnings and more in a big hurry. It was the action; I didn't care about the money in those days."

In fact, Arnie cared about little in those days. He was even blind to the fault lines about to sever his marriage. The inevitable divorce "didn't faze" him. "My gambling got worse. I did not have to account to anyone any more, I only had to account to myself." Even Arnie could not avoid the obvious: "This of course was another of my bad ideas, especially when I was drinking; the more I drank the more I didn't care how much money I lost—until the next day."

Arnie described a snappish barroom conversation when a friend advised him "how dumb" it was to lose $800 gambling. "I'd tell him that it was my money. And my business. Then the next day I'd think, 'What a dumb thing to do.'"

Arnie descended to rock bottom—twice. "When I had sixty days to move out of my apartment I started looking around for another place," Arnie recalls. "I was shocked that no one would rent to me because of my bad credit." The first of his rescuers appeared on the scene, a brother-in-law. "John sent me a check for $2,000, enough to pay 2-3 months on a new place to live." But Arnie's rational self was not yet in charge. The cash was taken straight to the casino and vanished at the poker table. After losing his house, car, an IRA ($2000) and John's rescue funds, Arnie got very drunk. Paradoxically, that's when reality set in.

The man who once hunted with his family now would turn the gun on himself. The only thing standing between himself and death was a phone call he placed to his sister in Napa. "She did the right thing," Arnie recalls. "She called the sheriff. They sent an ambulance and took me to the hospital." Brother-in-law John now upped the ante on Arnie's endowment, paying out more than $7,000 for an alcohol treatment program. After being in the treatment program for a few weeks and "learning about my addictions," Arnie concluded that "gambling was the worst."

The local Gambling Anonymous chapter had much to offer Arnie. But still he saw how easy it was to get sidetracked. "My nephew was paying a visit and he wanted to go to the casino," Arnie recalled. "I told him I'd just wait for him. But he insisted that I play $20. He said it was his money, not mine." Arnie watched the $20 vanish—followed by $1200 of his own."

There was an interval of five months between that casino night and a "gambling free" Arnie. But he knows staying clean is no sure thing. In fact, his days at GA meetings have given him new insights.

"I've seen 'em come (to meetings) because someone told them to come," he says. "But they won't quit. They won't stop until they're down in the gutter. College kids come here, after losing money they got to pay for schooling. But you can look at them and tell. They have no idea what this disease is all about."

Arnie, however, is an expert. Had his realizations about the "gambling gene" come earlier, he might have gravitated toward the health care field. GA meetings allow him to do the next best thing: recognize the scourge and try to warn the victim.

Chapter 22

The Bingo Addict:
Althea (age 49)

Troubled gamblers are reluctant to permanently give up an activity that serves as an important source of excitement and camaraderie in their lives.

—Martin C. McGurrin

ALTHEA'S HINDSIGHT SHOCKS HER STILL. During the throes of gambling addiction, she scammed friends, mistreated her children, and ignored her husband. "The lunacy of it," she says from a safe place.

Althea spent more time in church than most preachers. Sometimes she actually prayed—for a winning bingo number. One memorable prayer for cash was answered. "Please God," Althea had urged, "let some money come my way." As if from on high, the department store Macy's sent her a "refund" check for $190. Ecstatic, Althea took her windfall to the bingo parlor—and blew it. "Sometime later," Althea recalled, "Macy's sent a letter saying the check was issued in error. They put some kind of penalty on me."

Macy's, like many of Althea's creditors, was not likely to get their money soon. "On any given day," Althea says, "I was broke after a night of gambling." She was forced to take action. "I devised some very creative banking methods," Althea says, her voice tinged with gallows humor. "People would loan me money, and I'd write them a check. Then I'd put a stop on the check. You can only work that once with friends." She would then tell the friend it was a "mistake" and pay them back with money that had been borrowed elsewhere. It was her own private "pyramid scheme" and it left her filled with self-loathing. "People got wise to me," she says. "Or they at least suspected I was cheating them. And they were right." Althea tells her tale with the laughter of someone still incredulous about her behavior. "I had access to cash on my job. I'd convinced myself that I was only 'borrowing' and that after a big score I'd repay it. But the big score never came."

How did this spindly "silent, obedient child" from a large dysfunctional family wind up in the shady world of fundraising to feed her gambling addiction? It began innocently enough. "I guess it really started when I was a child," Althea said. "My brothers showed me how to pitch pennies. We'd actually slide them on the floor. Closest to the wall would win. I remember the nice thrill I'd get when I won. That's what stands out—the thrill. It was for sport—not winning the money." Later on, there were the occasional trips to Reno. "I played the slots, some blackjack, but it wasn't a serious problem." Althea admits that the fast action of blackjack and craps held no fascination for her.

That would happen later, when Althea turned 30. She had a family—a husband and two young children who counted on her. They struggled financially, but managed to provide necessities. But still there was a piece missing to Althea's puzzle. "I had never found a passion in my life," she says philosophically. "A lot of what I've read about compulsive gambling says it happens because people aren't pursuing what they love to do in life. They need to be doing something positive, something that is good for your psyche. I felt I had not found it."

That all changed swiftly. Althea's addiction came neatly wrapped, disguised as a charity.

"A friend told me about a local boys' club that had bingo on Tuesday nights. It was so innocent. A good cause. We'd be helping the children."

But Althea never dreamed that while "helping the children" she'd be destroying herself. "It just felt good when they called the numbers. Not to have your mind on other things. Not having to have your mind dwell on the realities of life. Plus you were out among a bunch of people. We all seemed to be having fun."

Tuesday night games blossomed into nightly occurrences. Althea, meanwhile, blossomed into the classic "escape-relief" gambler. This type of gambler describes it as "zoning out." Plus, there's that fantasy of the big win and the illusion that this will "square you" with all creditors.

"Bingo was popping up everywhere," Althea recalls. "You could always find a game. On a typical night, I'd lose about $100." But the worst of it all, for Althea, was how she "short-changed" her children. "They were forced to buy from second-hand stores. I'd skip giving them their allowance. I'd just piss it away gambling. I didn't like it. It was an uneasy feeling. You never know how you're going to rationalize these things. Mine was that I was going to make it up to them. I'd have a big win."

Althea retains a host of gambling-related memories—all painful. "Not so much the pain I've done to myself," she says. "It's the pain to others. Especially to my children." Althea's addiction was on the upswing when she discovered an afternoon bingo game that began at 1 p.m. "I thought I could leave the game in time to pick my kids up at school at 3:15. I'd be rushing like mad to their school, trying to rub the ink daubers off my hands. They'd ask where I'd been and I'd have to lie. One day I got there late . . . they were the only kids standing in the playground. In the sweltering heat."

Althea gets teary recalling one night when she was hurrying off to a bingo game and her daughter, then 7, blocked her way at the door. "Mommy, please stay home," the child said. Althea is stunned now at her own behavior: "I pushed her out of the way. Verrrry dramatic! But I had to get to the game."

By then Althea's gambling habit had ensnared her. She felt powerless. In addition to bingo, she indulged in keno and "scratchers." She'd shop at flea markets to save money for gambling. She cut back on quality food; her life was a whirlwind of rationalizations and racing to the next gambling venue. A stark clue to the magnitude of her addiction came when Althea found herself cashing in a life insurance policy.

"The lunacy of it," she says now from the relative safety of recovery. "There's no deceiving yourself. It's an emotional illness. It's compulsive behavior. It could have manifested itself in any way."

Althea's husband showed up several times at the bingo parlor, urging her to come home. Still compulsive, Althea thought "he was bringing me bad luck. There's an aspect of me that wants to be in control. Let me pull the trigger."

Now clean, Althea will likely spend a lifetime trying to make things up to her children, now adults. "I'll never really be able to make it up to them," she says earnestly. Althea had always hoped that her own family would be totally unlike what she had experienced as a child.

"My father always worked and was always unhappy," she recalled. "He was abusive; there was violence in the house. He was also vulgar. My father was incapable of being a person someone would want to have a chat with." Althea's siblings sought escape in their own addictions—drugs and alcohol. One is now in recovery. Althea's mother absorbed the family pain but then as an older adult went to college and started out on a new life. "I surely respect her for that," Althea says.

With her life under control—five years since her last gambling session—Althea has turned introspective about the addiction that once dragged her down to the nether world. "Once you identify yourself as a compulsive gambler, there is no going back," she says. "You're either a recreational gambler or a compulsive gambler. You can't be both."

Althea remembers vividly her first night in Gamblers Anonymous, responding to the organization's "20 questions." A few "yes" answers indicate a gambling problem. "I answered yes to all of them!"

About the national craze for gambling, Althea feels sympathy for those who won't remain recreational gamblers. "So many people are using it as their fix. The people you see in GA are just the top of the island you see above the water." Althea's luck came in the form of a husband who stuck with her and children still in the process of forgiveness.

Will Althea ever gamble again? She chuckles, quoting the Willy Nelson lyric, "I'd have to be crazy/plum out of my mind." Althea monitors the gambling surge in her own community. "We recently had a suicide over a $1500 gambling debt." At a rap group for teenagers, Althea talked about gambling problems among the young. "This one Asian girl talked about the gambling in her family. Both of her parents gambled. I was thinking at the time, 'Thank goodness my husband doesn't gamble too.' I could see how hard that was for this girl. That would have completely undone my children." As for the numbers of compulsive and problem gamblers in the nation—which the "gaming" industry puts at less than two percent—Althea is in total disagreement: "We don't even have a clue how many compulsive gamblers are out there ruining their lives."

Chapter 23

The Comic: Morrie (age 57)

For full-time gamblers, time loses much more than its context at the track. Post time is one. Tuesdays are dark. What else matters"
—Brendan Boyd

MORRIE'S LUNCHTIME GUESTS ONCE INCLUDED THE ENTIRE 1958 OFFENSIVE LINE of the Green Bay Packers. Translation: Morrie had raised "padding the expense account" to an art form. Other times he took the New York Yankees—"Tony Kubek, Billy Martin and Moose Skowron. We had a great time." Morrie favored double-play combinations as his imaginary dining companions. It spiked the ruse with a bit of irony, since the pilfered funds were wagered on some of these same athletes. "Wagers," Morrie says with sincere recollection, "usually made on the wrong team."

Morrie retains his New York accent. He's a West Coast transplant with fond memories of the East and even fonder memories of Gamblers Anonymous "rooms," as he calls them, "on both coasts and one, briefly, in the Midwest."

Morrie's slide into compulsive gambling is not unique. His mannerisms and taste for irony could have landed him in New York's Borscht Belt doing his shtick on stage, but he's dead serious when talking about the pain of addiction.

"Uncle Bernie was my favorite relative," Morrie says, recalling his early childhood. "I had no doubt that he was a compulsive gambler. He'd drive from Miami to New York, straight through, no sleep, and get a ticket in every state. There was always series of warrants out for him. He lived a very colorful life."

Morrie's own parents were less flamboyant than Uncle Bernie, gainfully employed and good providers. "My father gambled a little," Morrie says. "A friendly poker game. Nothing too serious." Family values were instilled early: "They definitely taught me right from wrong," Morrie says. "But once I started gambling compulsively, I didn't know right from wrong anymore."

The New York neighborhood kids flipped baseball cards, bet on stickball games, pitched pennies, and even placed fifty cent wagers on one block's baseball team taking on another. Morrie recalls "playing hookie, going to a kid's house and starting a poker game."

School held no interest. But Morrie's first big victory did. The young gamblers sneaked up to the roof of his brownstone on a summer night and played cards until 3 a.m. "I wiped everybody out," Morrie says gleefully. "I had all this change loading me down. My pockets were bulging." His parents were waiting up. "Boy did I get my ass whipped when they saw me coming in." But this was merely a temporary setback for Morrie's chosen lifestyle.

His first after-school job led to a rude awakening. "I brought home my first paycheck," he says. "And I thought my father would be proud." Instead, Morrie's father asked for the check. "Why?" protested Morrie.

"Do you live here?" Morrie's father asked.

"Yes."

"Do you pay rent?"

"No."

"Do you eat your meals here?"

"Yes."

"Do you pay for your meals?"

Morrie quickly got the point. He turned over his paychecks "to the household," but not without resentment. (Years later, when he was ready for college, Morrie would discover that the money had been put away for his education.)

Still in his teens, Morrie got his initiation to horse racing when some friends suggested a trip to Yonkers Raceway. "I worked in a day camp and some of the older guys went to the track frequently. They'd pick me up and I'd go along. It was my introduction to parimutuel betting." In essence, Yonkers was Morrie's launchpad into the capricious world of gambling: "It kept going from there. A chosen lifestyle."

Morrie had a five-year gap between high school and college, some of it spent working in a print shop, most of it spent gambling—horses, cards, sports betting, casinos. Any place there was action.

Morrie's boss at the print shop had a system for picking horses and was willing to share it. "It was based on the number of the winner of the previous race," Morrie says, slightly embarrassed. "But I tried it for several weeks, without betting. And it won consistently." But the first time Morrie plunked down a wager the inevitable happened: "It didn't work. And the idea was to double your bet when you lost."

Sounding like a Damon Runyon character, Morrie confesses: "I proceeded to drop a large chunk of money." Morrie seems plucked from that race track fraternity, a camaraderie of desperate loners seeking the monster payoff. Tips on horses are sought, praised, debunked and occasionally reach the finish wire first. The "racetrack tout" reached its apotheosis with the Marx Brothers in *A Day at the Races*—Groucho the sucker and Chico selling him not merely a tip but a stack of books, graphs and charts to crack the code that will reveal the winner. Morrie and thousands of others could attest to the fact that although the gag is spiked, the truth resonates. (Damon Runyon stories are packed with such touts, most notably "The Lemon Drop Kid," played in the movie version by a young Bob Hope.)

Morrie briefly abstained from the track and thrust himself into "higher education." Although the first day of college usually means orientation, textbooks, syllabi and the like, Morrie had his own plan. "I missed the first two weeks of school because I was up in the dorm playing poker," he says. "One long game. People would come and go. There was only one constant in the game—me." After two weeks, Morrie thought "wait a minute: I should go to a class. I'd walk in and they'd say 'who's this guy?' I didn't do well my first semester."

Although he managed a bachelor's degree in economics, Morrie was seduced by the illusion that he could make a living at gambling. "I thought about it many times," he says. "A friend and I used to go to Belmont Park. Our plan was to quit our jobs and then go on to Hialeah for the season. We thought it would be great. We'd sleep on the beach."

The plan never materialized, but Morrie found that gambling was beginning to consume all his waking hours. And it also led to less than honest behavior. "If someone wanted me to place a bet for them at the track, I'd be happy to take it. If they won I'd keep the winnings. Tell them I couldn't get the bet down and give them back their original bet. If they lost, I'd give them the losing ticket." Did Morrie have qualms about such behavior? "I should have. But I didn't. I'd do whatever I had to get money. I had to stay in action."

With a "clarity of mind" Morrie acquired only since he quit gambling, he says of his peak gambling period: "If I won every cent in the world I would give somebody money to play against me just so I can be in action. It was pointless. I would sit at a poker table with a losing hand and throw money in. It's only chips. It's just plastic."

These days Morrie speaks frequently of "seeing things with a clear mind," an impossible perspective when you're stuck in gambling addiction. Although his last bet was more than twenty years ago—as is typical of gamblers, Morrie can recall every detail of the losing wager—he attends his GA meetings religiously. He's often a mentor to those fresh off the gambling treadmill. The "expense account" memoir often brings a laugh to the listener. "It's something I tell new GA people when they're down in the dumps," Morrie says. "'You can't beat yourself up,' I tell him. 'You didn't do it because you were a bad person. You did it because you were a sick person.'"

In Morrie's case, he had to disabuse himself of the notion that "I'll do better at gambling once I learn to manage my money," or "I'm just having a bad streak." The ultimate wakeup call was loud and clear: "I got evicted from my apartment. I had been living without heat, phone or lights. I needed that money to gamble with. I reasoned that the landlord had so many units in the building he wouldn't miss it if I didn't pay the rent."

Friends helped convince Morrie he had "a serious gambling problem."

The first words Morrie heard from the GA counselor were succinct: "If you want to quit, you've made your last bet."

Morrie's retort: "How much would you put on that?"

But the sponsor did not laugh. "He looked at me," Morrie recalls, "and read me the riot act. This is a serious program. My landlord had just evicted me and some guy is telling me this ain't no joke. It was a real eye opener."

Twenty years in various GA programs have made Morrie something of an authority. "It goes something like this," Morrie says: "Work a hard (GA) program, have an easy recovery. Work an easy program, have a hard recovery." Morrie feels fortunate that he worked a hard program. "I have never gone back to gambling." But he's seen others in easier, less demanding programs who have foundered and felt that they could "gamble a little" but wound up back in the throes of addiction. What would Morrie say to those who think they can quit gambling without GA?

"I don't proselytize," Morrie notes. "I let them know there is a place where they can get help if they want the chance to live a normal happy life. But you have to be ready for it. You can't force anybody. They have to want to quit."

Chapter 24

A Hero's Spouse:
Mitzi (age 41)

*The (gambling addiction) high comes in escaping reality and believing
that past debts can be repaid quickly and effortlessly.*
—Dr. Valerie Lorenz

MITZI'S ANGUISH AND HEARTBREAK WERE PLAYED OUT IN PUBLIC. Husband Art
Schlichter was an Ohio State quarterback of epic skills. He signed on with
the Baltimore Colts in 1982 for a cash bonus of $350,000 and a salary of
$140,000—all of which he promptly gambled away. The NFL suspended
Art for a year, then reinstated him in 1984. That same year the couple met
on a blind date, Mitzi a senior at Ball State University in Indiana.

She had been raised a Catholic, had no exposure to gambling and had
no idea who Art was. The football hero was forthright enough to mention
his gambling problem. But, Mitzi recalls, Art put it in the "past tense." The
truth about Art's gambling addiction would astound even most compulsive gamblers. He wagered his salary as well as money he didn't have. His
NFL career ended abruptly in 1986, when the league banned him for life.
Now he would scramble not on the football field but in futile attempts to
raise more and more money to recoup losses. His sports prowess gave him
entrée to otherwise unavailable lines of credit. Bookies cut him slack. Art's
craving for gambling action was limitless. Explained his psychologist, Dr.

Valerie Lorenzi, "The high comes in escaping reality and believing that past debts can be repaid quickly and effortlessly."

Mitzi hung in for almost a decade of marriage, protecting her two young daughters from the sting of an absent father with an inexplicable illness. It was an endless cycle, Mitzi recalls. She was trying to figure out what was going on—suspicions she could not prove. She suffered anxiety, confusion, strange phone calls and conversations with Art that escalated into huge fights. Art sought help but continued gambling. Mitzi saw her husband as a tormented individual. They were divorced in 1998.

Art spent the next several years gambling, stealing, pleading, hustling and festering in prison. The press feasted on his misbegotten life, then forgot him. Schlichter was last heard from in the Marion County, Indiana, jail awaiting sentencing for theft, forgery and corrupt business influence for bilking nine people out of $250,000 and never giving them promised basketball tickets. He even got his attorney suspended after she smuggled a cell phone into prison in 2000 so Art could place bets.

Early on, Mitzi could have comforted herself through denial. Instead she has devoted herself to understanding the disease of gambling. She helped found the Custer Gambling Treatment Center in Indianapolis. When the National Gambling Impact Study Commission sought her testimony, Mitzi obliged. She even appeared on a TV talk show in Washington state, explaining how gambling can destroy individuals—and families.

Mitzi is charitable in her assessment of her ex-husband: "I know he has caused a lot of people pain," she told an Indianapolis newspaper reporter, "and I've felt very angry at him, just like everybody has. But at the same time, I know his pain is also very real. That's been hard to watch. The most painful thing about the process is seeing the turmoil he's been in for such a long time. He's very sick, and I think he needs a lot of help."

Mitzi and her daughters, now 15 and 11, have moved beyond the family trauma. But she has heartfelt empathy for families of compulsive gamblers. She knows about empty promises and rent money used to pay off bookies. About husbands declaring that they can fix the financial problems.

Mitzi urges families to come forward and seek help, even if the gambler is in recovery. She advises wives of compulsive gamblers to safeguard themselves by signing nothing jointly—no checking accounts, loans or credit cards. Mitzi realizes that wives are often convinced they need their gambling husband to survive. But, she counsels from experience, "once you've left the relationship most of your financial problems will be gone as well."

Part 4

THE LAST ACT

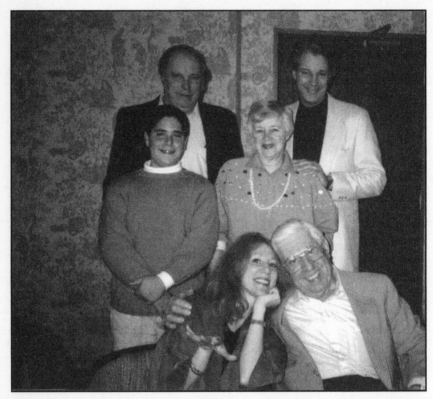

Phil Dragin (front right) marks 80th birthday in Las Vegas with (top) his sons Bill and Burt, Mark (Bill's son), Fae Dragin and (front left) Nadine, after her performance as Adelaide with Burt as Nathan Detroit from Guys and Dolls.

Chapter 25

A Milestone

The 1990s rushed by like a thoroughbred under the skilled hands of jockey Willie Shoemaker.

By THE 1990s MY PARENTS WERE FIRMLY ENSCONCED in a retirement community called Murrieta, north of San Diego. All the amenities were present except for a casino. "I tried making book," my father told me. "Guys make a few bets. They lose. So they quit." He settled for gin rummy and poker at the clubhouse. The mortality rate of the senior residents was predictable. "When a guy drops out of a hand," my father quipped, "you may never see him again."

There was betting action nearby, though. On one of his periodic trips to Off Track Betting at nearby Perris, my father plunked down one dollar and played the "Pick 8" at Hollywood Park racetrack. He held one of five winning tickets, good for a tidy $3,853. My parents bought a big-screen TV and the rest vanished at Pechanka, an Indian casino "9.5 miles away, door to door."

In 1992 my father marks a milestone, his eightieth birthday, celebrated in—where else? My wife Nadine and I fly to Vegas rehearsing our tribute—banter from *Guys & Dolls* embellished to include the notorious gambler Phil Dragin. The venue is my folks' hotel room. As Dad is seated, surrounded by Mom, Bill, his wife Judy and youngest son Mark, Nadine and I, as Adelaide and Nathan Detroit (in appropriate garb), perform:

NATHAN: Boy Adelaide, can you believe the action in this town? And the players who showed up!

ADELAIDE: Who Nathan?

NATHAN: Why, The Greek's in town. And Brandy Bottle Bates. And Scranton Slim. And get this: Phil Dragin!

ADELAIDE: Phil Dragin of Cleveland?

NATHAN: That's the one.

ADELAIDE: Phil Dragin of Amato's Pool Hall, and The Mystics and the Norwalk Trucking Company?

NATHAN: The same.

ADELAIDE: What's he doing in Vegas?

NATHAN: He's celebrating his birthday. He often comes to Vegas to celebrate things.

ADELAIDE: Like what else?

NATHAN: Well, last month he came here to celebrate...Tuesday!

ADELAIDE: You know, Nathan, I hear that Phil Dragin is the guy who put Pete Maroni where he is today?

NATHAN: No kidding. By the way Adelaide, where is Pete Maroni today?

ADELAIDE: I hear he's partners in a pig farm in Acapulco!

My father takes great delight in the performance. He's a mixture of laughter and tears, suffused in nostalgia.

Then Nadine, in costume, does her marvelous "Adelaide's Lament" and brings down the house. Now Nadine and I can say we "played" Vegas.

Had my father beaten the 6 to 5 odds of which all life is against? A life-long compulsive gambler, in his eighties, he was in decent physical health, married, and owned a home, free and clear, and bills paid on time. Or was he in purgatory? "Your mother gives me $50 a week allowance," he says in his now raspy voice. "If I blow it I have no money to gamble until the next week. Then I have nothing to do." It's his common refrain. I never know how to reply.

"Still," he says, "your mother put up with me all these years. That's something." It's clear from his tone that my father is doing penance. My mother controls the cash and therefore rules the roost. My father, sadly, is frequently less than lucid. His talk is splattered with unfinished sentences, obscure references and a plaintive, repetitious: "My problem was that no one ever told me what was what."

The 1990s rushed by like a thoroughbred under the skilled hands of jockey Willie Shoemaker. Meanwhile, I'm still playing gumshoe in the world of gambling addiction research. Below the surface my own craving for action has returned. This produces a conflicted state of mind. I'm seeking the cause, and nursing the yen.

I complete a phone interview with gambling researcher Dr. Richard Rosenthal and he asks if I'm attending the annual conference of the National Council on Problem Gambling. "Where? When?" I ask him. The conference is two weeks away—in Las Vegas. To reduce temptation, the three-day conference is held at the Alexis Park Resort, the only major Vegas hotel without a casino.

(As I'm writing this, the phone rings. It's Jack, telling me I've been "selected for a special Reno promotion. Three days, two nights and $70 in cash to gamble. All for $99." Pause. "I'm a compulsive gambler." I had never said it before; I wondered how Jack would react. "Well," he says, undismayed, "you don't have to gamble.")

Chapter 26

Snake Bit

I'm at the crap table, watching my stack of chips reduced to nothing.

I DECIDE TO ATTEND THE NATIONAL COUNCIL ON PROBLEM GAMBLING CONFER-
ENCE, and strategically book my Las Vegas flights: airport to conference,
conference to airport and home. The Alexis Park Resort lobby is teeming
with gambling research celebrities; hawkers of books, pamphlets, audio
tapes; clinicians of every stripe; curious hotel guests; and some Vegas
casino execs who represent their establishments "in an unceasing quest to
eradicate compulsive gambling" (or so they would have us believe).

I scan the program and am overwhelmed with the choices, sev-
eral sessions per time slot. Psychiatrists, psychologists, researchers and
authors will discuss "Typology of Pathological Gamblers," "Gambling
Among Seniors," "Responsible Gaming and the Lottery," "Spirituality
and Gambling: Cultural Predispositions," "Minorities and Gambling
Treatment," "Psychodrama and Compulsive Gambling," "Impact of
Gambling Problems on the Family," "Excessive Gambling Among
Adolescents," "Interactive Gambling."

I mark my choices and purchase a raft of audio tapes. I spend two days frantically taking notes, making contacts and gleaning all I can about an addiction whose shrines are just blocks away on the Vegas Strip. Where would I rather be? The answer isn't encouraging.

Throughout the sessions I hear several reference to "sogs"; "sogs this" and "sogs that" and I'm too embarrassed to ask. Finally I learned that it's SOGS—South Oaks Gambling Screen, a 16-question survey devised in 1992 that determines if you're a compulsive gambler.

On the final day of the conference I'm guzzling coffee while moderator Mark Hagwood presents "The Lessons of History," which includes a fetching chapter called "The Wild Wild West: Gambling on the Old Frontier." I'm intrigued through this entire session, which—to my surprise—ends abruptly. Blinding florescent lights are flicked on. The conference is over! It's only 1:30 pm. My flight is at 7 tonight—I have miscalculated by several hours.

I climb into my rental car and sit, ignoring the magnetism of The Strip for as long as I can. Minutes later I'm sitting down at a moderate stakes Hold 'Em poker game at the Stardust Hotel. It's a way to ride out the time, provided the cards prove agreeable. They don't. I pick up stiff hand after stiff hand. My stomach muscles tighten.

Next I'm at the crap table, watching my stack of chips reduced to nothing. "Snake bit," I think. What to do? Take a later flight? Punch up the ATM machine? Here I am in the lion's den, the expert voices from the last 48 hours thick in my consciousness. I feel the tug of the dice table, tempting me to get even. My watch shows it's time to get to the airport, return the rental car, and make the flight. But I'm mesmerized by clanging slots, players' chatter, and green felt. I reach for my wallet and extract the ATM card; my pulse races.

This is laughable, I think. I start to weaken, then my mind is pierced by a thought that rarely troubles the true compulsive gambler—what if I lose even more? The next day is Father's Day, which I want to spend with my wife Nadine and our daughter Ana—and my self-esteem intact. I know the consequences if this trip turns into a major fiasco. I picture myself chasing the losses all night, arriving home Sunday ashen-faced and ashamed. I've seen it happen to too many compulsive gamblers. Their images appear in my mind like a Greek chorus, intoning my fate. Silently I thank them and make the flight.

The next day I ruminate in self-analysis. Prognosis: I am caught between the passion to gamble and the red flags that pop up when I head for the casino. An initial losing streak is what does me in—a maddening loss of self-esteem that veers into self-flagellation. From there I can only recoup myself by recouping my chips. More losses equal more anguish. It's a familiar story. And as Indian casinos bloom closer to my home turf I feel more and more vulnerable.

The Vegas trip to the NCPG, I decided, was an anomaly. When else would a compulsive gambler hit the casino with such psychic baggage— that is, a head full of dire warnings of disaster? The gods have cooked up another Las Vegas trip and one more chance to inhale the heady ether of risk.

My odyssey has begun seeping into my unconscious. As I write this book, gambling dreams are common. In surreal Dali-esque casinos, I'm frantically searching for a crap table. Sometimes I find one with a dozen dice in play; other times as I approach the crap table it morphs into an unrecognizable shape.

Chapter 27

Seventy Years!

Back to the poker machines; man and machines, no screw-ups.

It's the big "Fae and Phil 70th anniversary," and my parents, of course, choose Las Vegas as the venue. I figure I'm bound to win, the karma on my side, since I did not choose the destination. (Gamblers look for signs anywhere.) Of course, I don't protest a Vegas trip. That's sacrilege. We're all booked into the Golden Nugget downtown, ten of us.

You'd think we'd celebrate at a dinner show, but this is strictly a gambling trip—a few family meals, and you're on your own. Soon our original family of four are pumping quarters into the poker machines. My father hits four-of-a-kind three times in the first hour, each good for 200 bucks.

I'm sipping a beer and musing about the throngs of people battling the house edge. I conclude that I understand compulsive gamblers and professional gamblers but cannot fathom "recreational" gamblers. These are the folks who lose their limit—$50 or $500—and stop. Such gamblers call this "entertainment." But for me, losing is a personal affront, a solid blow to my psyche that begs for retaliation. Which is why I shouldn't be here. But I'm clocked in for roughly 72 hours. Several beers help lubricate the encounter.

I cross Fremont Street and stride into Binyon's Horseshoe, scene of the World Series of Poker. Three months earlier a man with the unlikely name of Chris Moneymaker startled the poker world by winning Binion's annual World Series of Poker, pocketing $2.5 million. This unknown 27-year-old had skewered the poker elite. Moneymaker got into the tournament by investing a mere $40 and winning several online poker tournaments. (The normal World Series of Poker entry fee is $10,000.) Moneymaker's victory sparked a nationwide craze in Texas Hold 'Em. Online poker sites blossomed. Cable TV's Travel Channel cashed in with the *World Poker Tour* while ESPN screened the *World Series of Poker* in various installments, along with *Celebrity Poker.* Television also launched a spate of casino dramas, most notably *Las Vegas,* starring James Caan, whose portrayal of Axel Freed in *The Gambler* (1975) was the purest cinematic rendition of a compulsive gambler. Caan's return in *Las Vegas* as Big Ed Deline, a former CIA agent now in charge of Vegas casino security, is TV fare of the most contrived and vapid sort.

At Binion's I manage to win about $300 in Hold 'Em. But in the course of the game, after being crushed in a major pot I'm fuming as I stride blindly toward the men's room. I slap the wall in a spontaneous gesture of futility. ("What happened to your hand," my daughter asks the next morning. I'm shocked to see that my entire palm has turned purple.)

By the next night at the Nugget I feel compelled to square off at the crap table. Awareness of why I may be doing this makes it no less appealing. Let the dopamine rip! Indulge my genetic birthright! Regress to infantile megalomania! Who cares about the adult world?

I pick up the dice and make pass after pass. The trim blond on my left is elated, sharing high fives each time I hit a point. I down a fresh beer, watching my chips grow like a snake on the wooden rail. I'm even betting (and hitting) the hard ways! "Two-way hard ten," I yell, indicating I'm making a bet for the dealers. How gorgeous life can be! These red cubes are magic! My students would be shocked. Their laid-back journalism professor screaming, clapping his hands, ecstatic!

Then I feel disaster on my right. It's my father. He's peeling a wad of bills. When he was younger, say 80, he'd never walk in during my roll. It's the classic crap shooter's superstition. You're on fire, dice under control, then someone moves in to tilt the universe a thread and the streak dies. *Never* fails. Never! "Just a minute," I whisper. "Let me make this pass." I'm really pissed—and conflicted. How can I shun my father on his 70th anniversary? Yet I wish he'd never walked up. I make the point—five.

Now my father's dropping a ten dollar bill on the green felt, calling a $30 bet. He must have thought it was a hundred; he's confused, squinting through his thick glasses. The pit boss and dealers are chuckling. I'm pained. A poor requiem for a lifetime crapshooter. The other players are wincing; my streak has no chance. My father fumbles with the green bills. "What?" he asks the dealers. "What?" They explain he called a bet but didn't put down enough money. I glance at my father. He looks all of his 91 years. Players are leaving the table. Eventually, the game resumes. I pick up the dice and promptly crap out, trying to make a six.

"Want me to leave?" my father asks.

"Let's both go," I say. The beers help drown out my shame and sadness over time's heartless theft of my father's mental faculties. Back to the poker machines; man and machine, no screw-ups. More beer. More quarters to pump into eternity. I do manage to avoid my prime fear—chasing. Fortunately, I never have to reach for the ATM card. Actually, I come out slightly ahead. In money. But emotionally, I lose a ton. It happens hours before my flight. One last meal together. My father is missing from the dining area, and I go off to search in the casino, dodging through the mirrors, the glitz, peering down rows of poker machines. Players are sipping coffee, smoking. Casino action during the afternoon has always struck me as unnatural, depressing.

No luck. I return to the restaurant. No one knows where he is. "He may be lost," says my mother. "Let me go look. I know what shirt he's wearing." Meanwhile, my father had secured us a table in another part of the restaurant, and there he sits, alone. I approach and tell him that Mom went to look for him. He gets up to go find her. "No," I say. "Stay at our table. I'll take care of it." My father is suddenly livid. Then it happens.

"You don't take care of nothing."

"What?"

"You heard me," he says. His face is boiling. "You don't do nothing for me. You're the cheapest son of a bitch I ever met in my life."

It's his best shot. In my father's pantheon of miscreants the cheapskate is one notch above the axe murderer.

"But," I stammer in astonishment, still operating on the last beer, "I offered to send you some gambling money each month. You said not to."

"That's not the way to do it." Evidently, he was afraid Mom would discover my letters with checks in them. Bill, it turns out, slips him the cash. Bill lives an hour away, visits him frequently. I live in the goddamn Bay Area. My father continues.

"All my friends tell me 'how generous your son Bill is.'" He rambles on, praising Bill, belittling me. He's really into it, spitting venom.

I'm stunned, hurt and angry, but I find my voice.

"Well," I say, "at least you got one good son. That's batting five hundred. Five hundred's pretty good." I'm saying empty words, stifling a counterattack.

"Damned right," he says. He'd once spent a whole weekend introducing me to his buddies as his "college professor son" and now this. Had he just lost the rest of his stake? Is he attacking me instead of striking the wall?

Phil's always been Mr. Happy-Go-Lucky. At least on the outside.

Finally all the family members are seated and we eat. I'm in shock, unable to look at my father. The food is tasteless.

I pick up the tab, refusing to let Bill contribute. My father gives me a limp "thank you."

"My pleasure," I hear myself saying, aching inside.

Chapter 28

Faux Addiction?

Once again I feel trapped between the gambling urge and the potential for chasing losses into masochistic flameout.

BACK HOME TO MY SODDEN LIFE. Do I have something unique—faux addiction? And if so, what's the cure? I discover in my research, perhaps not coincidentally, a noted psychologist who specializes in compulsive gambling and sanctions treatment without total abstinence. "The practice may be questionable," writes Neil D. Isaacs, "but I cannot in good conscience rule out a resumption of gambling by a client for whom it may be manageable, pleasurable, affordable, and acceptable to spouse, family, colleagues, and employers."

Isaacs tacks on a load of provisos. The gambler must have:

(1) A sufficiently developed observing ego to be aware of changes in his own behavior;
(2) A clear understanding of the distinctions between habitual and pathological gambling;
(3) A well-placed warning system among family and friends about changes in his gambling;

(4) A demonstrated ability to be abstinent in response to warning
    signals;
(5) A comprehension of his own gambling nature and history that
    includes possible origins of the habit and possible triggers for cross-
    ing over the line into pathology; and, perhaps most important,
(6) No indication that the pathology has ever reached the point of
    addiction where any bet would trigger an uncontrollable escala-
    tion of action.

This strikes me as heartbreak for a gambler in treatment seeking even
the narrowest of paths back to the casino. He'd have to be heavily medi-
cated to abide by such constrictions, especially number six.

Once again I feel trapped between the gambling urge and the potential for chasing losses into masochistic flameout. Don't go there, a voice
says. Have I placed myself in recovery? But what of the urge, the constant
thoughts about gambling?

Then I find the gambler's methadone. At a cavernous discount furniture store in downtown Berkeley I am kibitzing with Larry, the owner. As
Nadine is checking out TV stands, Larry and I pierce the small talk and
find common ground: gambling. Larry's key words burst above his head
like tantalizing cartoon thought balloons: *Weekly poker game. Two hundred
dollar buy-in. Three raises. Five dollar limit. Ten dollars in draw.*

We exchange phone numbers. Six weeks later I'm a player. The games
are perfect; each player owns a green felt poker table and springs for a
meal. They even have a website, and players must RSVP. There's the usual
table talk—the male libido, sports, women, politics, women, but there's
also certified anger over being "gutted"—your apparent winning hand
nailed by an even better one. These games used to go all night, I'm told.
Now they stop around 1 a.m. I've been accepted as a "regular" although
the tag of "new guy" can stick for ten years.

Friday morning I'm looking forward to the next game. But there is a downside. At one game I drop three hundred plus and am strangled by the familiar anguish—pulse climbing, mind exploding, all rationality gone. If only, I think, if only this were a casino. I'd be at the crap table trying to recoup...what? The money? My equilibrium? Self esteem? The drive home has a calming effect. There are casinos nearby, but there is the class I must teach tomorrow, and there's always next week's game.

Thursdays arrive quickly, and I settle into my weekly "high." Sitting down at the green felt, two hundred dollars worth of chips and a string of beers is a giddy sensation. Each game a fresh start—endless possibilities stoked by risk and hope. And beneath the table talk this is a fiercely competitive poker game. I'm told winners have struck for over one thousand dollars. In my third game I witness a rush that nets the garrulous Norm over six hundred. And there are lessons here.

As the writer Somerset Maugham observed:

> The student of human nature can find endless matter for observation in the behavior of his fellow card players. Meanness and generosity, prudence and audacity, courage and timidity, weakness and strength—all these men show at the card table according to their natures, and because they are intent upon the game, they drop the mask they wear in the ordinary affairs of life.

For me the challenge is remaining calm after a bitterly lost hand; my impulse to fling the cards in the air and upturn the table must be squelched. It's no time to go into a rage. Being invited back—fitting in—is the most important thing. That rational I am. For the moment, I have the gambling compulsion in check. But those "Vegas weekend fling" ads are more than slightly tempting. And I quickly realize that a weekly game leaves me limp for the week. What about tacking on Monday night Hold 'Em sessions at a local Indian casino? That way I'll have no more than four days between action. I give it a try, lecturing myself on the drive out Highway 80 East: *you have a few hundred invested . . . you might win, you might lose . . . the cards fall at random . . . if I lose I lose . . . I won't get upset . . . I won't get upset.*

During the third Monday session I scrap all reason. I play two hours and don't take a hand. Worse, I drop out with hands that would have won. It's gut-wrenching action. You have a string of losses; then you drop out of a hand and watch the flop (three communal cards) followed by the fourth card (the "turn") and the final card (the "river"). Out of the hand, you don't have to watch. But I do, realizing that I've folded a winner. This becomes the pattern; stay in and get trounced, or drop with a winner. My pre-gambling lecture on rationality dissolves. My gut fills with bile; I hate everyone at the table, especially the guy on my left—peering over his mountain of chips—who seeks my sympathy when he loses one measly hand. I sneer at him. I toss in my last chip and get slammed even though I hold a strong pair. I'm finished. Blood pressure rising, I push myself up from the chair, ignoring players' stares.

Now I'm at the precipice. I head for the men's room, toss cold water in my face—avoiding my reflection. Where to? More cash? Back to the game? Then a forced glance in the mirror. God, I know this person. I *loathe* this person. I *will not* be this person. My mind is a pinwheel of conflicting desires. Get back in the game. Leave. The cards must change. Try another two hundred. Get even, then leave! Next comes the clincher, unbidden, from the depth of my consciousness: "It's a *drug,* you jerkoff." Out on the parking lot I'm met by a bracing wind whipping off the bay. On the ride home I'm a volcano, trying to hold it in. Then I explode, screaming obscenities like a junkie denied his fix.

Next morning in class I'm lecturing with a voice painfully hoarse. Later, sitting in my office, I mull over last night's insanity. I cop to Maeterlinck's term "puerile vanity." Or, as Dr. Isaacs would say, I'd slipped into an "uncontrollable escalation of action." Clearer still: I'd slipped into the skin of someone I *refuse* to be. I scrap the potentially tortuous Monday casino sessions and limit myself to the Thursday games.

Chapter 29

Final Thoughts

The unexamined life is not worth living—or wagering.

AND WHAT OF THOSE COMPULSIVE (AND PROBLEM) GAMBLERS who have not secured a safe substitute? What wisdom have I garnered on their behalf in years of research and observation? Clearly, gambling addiction can spring from a host of psychological "needs." It can vary in intensity and duration and—I'm certain—the diagnostic category "impulse control disorder" is no myth, despite the protestations of Dr. Vatz. But how do you know when you're truly hooked? Dr. Isaacs poses the key questions:

- When does the habit become a problem?

- When does the problem become pathology (illness)?

- If gamblers lie about their habit, how can they be afforded treatment?

- If gamblers lie to themselves, how can they acknowledge their problem?

- If full-blown pathology is required for diagnosis and treatment, won't it be too late to arrest or reverse the consequences of the condition?

In the annals of compulsive gambling literature, one would be hard pressed to find a story more tragic than that of Solomon Bell. He was a gambler clearly beyond the "consequences of his condition." It was only a matter of time. A Detroit police officer, Bell was off duty on January 26, 2000, and had lost several thousand dollars playing blackjack at the MGM Grand Detroit Casino.

He left the MGM and tried his luck at the Motor City Casino, where he again lost heavily. Then Bell tried a bold move, betting $4,000 on one hand. He was dealt a twenty but the dealer made 21. According to newspaper accounts, Bell screamed "No," took out his service revolver and shot himself in the head. He died instantly.

Solomon Bell was 38 and had been on the Oak Park force for 12 years. "This guy would be one of the last I'd ever guess would do something like this," commented a city official. "He was always on an even keel."

Bell's plight is hard to fathom. How does a man gamble himself to the point where he must obliterate his existence? Sadly, any compulsive gambler (and many problem gamblers) would have no trouble comprehending Solomon Bell's desperate act.

Those who find gambling simply a waste of time and money will never understand the addict. Yet many people hooked on gambling are encouraged by a society that worships riches. Our economic system has a simple playbook: "Get yours—any way you can." Headline coverage of lottery winners fuels the dream. Gambling may be the last—and worst—hope. Those of us seduced by its thrill factor must ask ourselves some questions:

- What are we ultimately willing to risk for the thrill?

- And what about those family members unwittingly along for the ride? What do they stand to gain—or lose?

Dr. Paul Good's observation is worth repeating: "A social gambler does not have any emotional investment in the outcome." So, if your psyche is elated or devastated by two tiny six-sided cubes falling randomly, you've got to wonder why. The answer may be revealing. To paraphrase Socrates: The unexamined life is not worth living—or wagering.

As I learned and have shared with you, there is no "typical" compulsive gambler. Mental states range from the desperation of Solomon Bell to the slender hope of Vincent (a pseudonym), whom I observed at a GA meeting in Palm Springs, California, where membership at the weekly meetings had jumped from about seven to thirty following the arrival of Indian casinos. There were the predictable stories of abstinence and anguish; temptation and acquiescence; taut nerves and release; and, of course, untold dollars tossed to the wind by an addiction that leaves no tracks.

There were gamblers clean for 25 years and others counting by days and hours. There were close to thirty people sharing the past, some beyond temptation, others with their demons in clear view.

But there was also Vincent sitting at table's end. It was his first meeting; he declined to speak and sat erect with fists clenched, emanating the pain of addiction and the bleak awareness that he would have the final word on his destiny.

What struck me about these GA members was the empathy in their comments directed toward Vincent. It wasn't "here's the warning, here's the consequences." It was a graceful acknowledgment of Vincent's plight and the tug-of-war seething in his brain.

The GA members allowed that "it may seem impossible now" but we've been there and there is a way out. But it's clearly a choice. Vincent absorbed it all but his body language was noncommittal.

In the midst of the "testimony" came an insight I had never before heard at GA, or anywhere else for that matter. I'm sure it was prompted by Vincent's presence. "There's a real shame one feels about being in GA at first," the member said. "But there's no shame in our society for being a gambler. It really should be just the opposite."

Two weeks later while conducting a telephone interview with a subject who had attended the meeting, I inquired hesitantly about Vincent. Had he fled GA for the casinos' false promise? No. Vincent had attended the very next GA meeting. Perhaps his fists had loosened up, and he was overcoming his shame.

And what about my father? We hadn't spoken since our confrontation in Vegas. I felt blameless and aggrieved. That he should have such a sordid opinion of me—even if unfounded—still hurts. I replay that restaurant scene over and over, wishing I could change the ending.

Then his 92nd birthday arrives. I send him a check for $100 and a copy of a 70-year-old photo my cousin Ruthe supplied me, showing Dad and his three brothers lined up in the back yard of their Cleveland home, his brother Ben on his right. My father is now the lone survivor. I know this photo will get his attention, but I don't know if he'll smile or wince. Or both. We speak by phone a few days later. He's upbeat, delighted with the photo. And extremely grateful for the $100 stake. "I don't know how I got so lucky to have two wonderful sons," he says. I thank him, relieved and grateful to hear his acknowledgment of me. Dad's suddenly engaging and lucid. We kibitz for a while.

Then it occurs to me: has he completely forgotten his "cheapest SOB I ever met" remark?

I'd bet on it.

Postscript: My father began his mental slide soon after my parents celebrated their 71st wedding anniversary. Forbidden to drive and without access to gambling action, he apparently had no reason to live. Senile dementia took over his mind, and he began to threaten my mother. She endured it all, offering love and support, all of it rejected. He died October 9, 2004.

Phil Dragin was sent to his eternal reward with a pair of dice in his breast coat pocket. He will never again feel the sting of a losing bet.

Resources

Gamblers Anonymous offers the following questions to anyone who may have a gambling problem. These questions are provided to help the individual decide if he or she is a compulsive gambler and wants to stop gambling.

TWENTY QUESTIONS

1. Did you ever lose time from work or school due to gambling?
2. Has gambling ever made your home life unhappy?
3. Did gambling affect your reputation?
4. Have you ever felt remorse after gambling?
5. Did you ever gamble to get money with which to pay debts or otherwise solve financial difficulties?
6. Did gambling cause a decrease in your ambition or efficiency?
7. After losing did you feel you must return as soon as possible and win back your losses?
8. After a win did you have a strong urge to return and win more?
9. Did you often gamble until your last dollar was gone?

10. Did you ever borrow to finance your gambling?

11. Have you ever sold anything to finance gambling?

12. Were you reluctant to use "gambling money" for normal expenditures?

13. Did gambling make you careless of the welfare of yourself or your family?

14. Did you ever gamble longer than you had planned?

15. Have you ever gambled to escape worry or trouble?

16. Have you ever committed, or considered committing, an illegal act to finance gambling?

17. Did gambling cause you to have difficulty in sleeping?

18. Do arguments, disappointments or frustrations create within you an urge to gamble?

19. Did you ever have an urge to celebrate any good fortune by a few hours of gambling?

20. Have you ever considered self-destruction or suicide as a result of your gambling?

Most compulsive gamblers will answer yes to at least seven of these questions.

SOUTH OAKS GAMBLING SCREEN (SOGS)

1. Please indicate which of the following types of gambling you have done in your lifetime. For each type, mark one answer: "not at all," "less than once a week" or "once a week or more."

	not at all	less than once a week	once a week or more	
a.	___	___	___	play cards for money
b.	___	___	___	bet on horses, dogs or other animals (at OTB, the track or with a bookie)
c.	___	___	___	bet on sports (parlay cards, with a bookie, or at Jai Alai)
d.	___	___	___	played dice games (including craps, over and under or other dice games) for money
e.	___	___	___	gambled in a casino (legal or otherwise)
f.	___	___	___	played the numbers or bet on lotteries
g.	___	___	___	played bingo for money
h.	___	___	___	played the stock, options and/or commodities maket
i.	___	___	___	played slot machines, poker machines or other gambling machines
j.	___	___	___	bowled, shot pool, played golf or some other game of skill for money
k.	___	___	___	pull tabs or "paper" games other than lotteries
l.	___	___	___	some form of gambling not listed above (please specify) _____

2. What is the largest amount of money you have ever gambled with on any one day?
   ___ never have gambled
   ___ $1 or less
   ___ more than $1 up to $10
   ___ more than $10 up to $100
   ___ more than $100 up to $1,000
   ___ more than $1,000 up to $10,000
   ___ more than $10,000

3. Check which of the following people in your life has (or had) a gambling problem.

___ father   ___ mother   ___ a brother or sister   ___ a grandparent

___ my spouse or partner   ___ my child(ren) ___ another relative

___ a friend or someone else important in my life

4. When you gamble, how often do you go back another day to win back money you lost?

___ never
___ some of the time (less than half the time I lost)
___ most of the time I lost
___ every time I lost

5. Have you ever claimed to be winning money gambling but weren't really? In fact, you lost?

___ never (or never gamble)
___ yes, less than half the time I lost
___ yes, most of the time

6. Do you feel you have ever had a problem with betting money or gambling?

___ no
___ yes, in the past but not now
___ yes

7. Did you ever gamble more than you intend to?

___ yes   ___ no

8. Have people criticized your betting or told you that you had a gambling problem, regardless of whether or not you thought it was true?

___ yes   ___ no

9. Have you ever felt guilty about the way you gamble or what happens when you gamble?

___ yes   ___ no

10. Have you ever felt like you would like to stop betting money or gambling but didn't think you could?

___ yes   ___ no

11. Have you ever hidden betting slips, lottery tickets, gambling money, I.O.U.s or other signs of betting or gambling from your spouse, children or other important people in your life?

___ yes   ___ no

12. Have you ever argued with people you live with over how you handle money?

___ yes   ___ no

13. (If you answered yes to question 12): Have money arguments ever centered on your gambling?

___ yes   ___ no

14. Have you ever borrowed from someone and not paid them back as a result of your gambling?

___ yes   ___ no

15. Have you ever lost time from work (or school) due to betting money or gambling?

___ yes   ___ no

16. If you borrowed money to gamble or to pay gambling debts, who or where did you borrow from? (check "yes" or "no" for each)

	no	yes
a. from household money	☐	☐
b. from your spouse	☐	☐
c. from other relatives or in-laws	☐	☐
d. from banks, loan companies or credit unions	☐	☐
e. from credit cards	☐	☐
f. from loan sharks	☐	☐
g. you cashed in stocks, bonds or other securities	☐	☐
h. you sold personal or family property	☐	☐
i. you borrowed on your checking account (passed bad checks)	☐	☐
j. you have (had) a credit line with a bookie	☐	☐
k. you have (had) a credit line with a casino	☐	☐

Scores on the SOGS are determined by adding up the number of questions
that show an "at risk" response.

Questions 1, 2 and 3 are not counted.

_____ Question 4 –   "most of the time I lose" OR "every time I lose"

_____ Question 5 –   "yes, less than half the time I lose" OR "every time
I lose"

_____ Question 6 –   "yes, in the past but not now" OR "yes"

_____ Question 7 –   "yes"

_____ Question 8 –   "yes"

_____ Question 9 –   "yes"

_____ Question 10 –   "yes"

_____ Question 11 –   "yes"

Question 12 – not counted

_____ Question 13 –   "yes"

_____ Question 14 –   "yes"

_____ Question 15 –   "yes"

_____ Question 16a –   "yes"

_____   b – "yes"

_____   c – "yes"

_____   d – "yes"

_____   e – "yes"

_____   f – "yes"

_____   g – "yes"

_____   h – "yes"

_____   i – "yes"

Questions 16j and k not counted

Total + _____ (there are 20 questions that are counted)

0 _ no problem
1–4 = some problem
5 or more = probable pathological gambler

©1992 South Oaks Foundation

NATIONAL GAMBLING IMPACT STUDY COMMISSION REPORT
Table 4-1: DSM-IV Criteria for Pathological Gambling

Preoccupation	Is preoccupied with gambling (e.g., preoccupied with reliving past gambling experiences, handicapping or planning the next venture, or thinking of ways to get money with which to gamble)
Tolerance	Needs to gamble with increasing amounts of money in order to achieve the desired excitement
Withdrawal	Is restless or irritable when attempting to cut down or stop gambling
Escape	Gambles as a way of escaping from problems or relieving dysphoric mood (e.g., feelings of helplessness, guilt, anxiety, or depression)
Chasing	After losing money gambling, often returns another day in order to get even ("chasing one's losses")
Lying	Lies to family members, therapists, or others to conceal the extent of involvement with gambling
Loss of control	Has made repeated unsuccessful efforts to control, cut back, or stop gambling
Illegal acts	Has committed illegal acts (e.g., forgery, fraud, theft) in order to finance gambling
Risked significant relationship	Has jeopardized or lost a significant relationship, job, or educational or career opportunity because of gambling
Bailout	Has relied on others to provide money to relieve a desperate financial situation caused by gambling

(Source: National Opinion Research Center at the University of Chicago, Gemini Research, and The Lewin Group. Gambling Impact and Behavior Study. Report to the National Gambling Impact Study Commission. April 1, 1999. Table 1, p. 16.)

Contacts

National Council on Problem Gambling
216 G Street, NE, 2nd Floor
Washington, DC 20002
Office: (202) 547-9204
Fax: (202) 547-9206
Helpline: 800.522.4700
ncpg@ncpgambling.org
www.ncpgambling.org
Executive director: Keith Whyte
Program Manager: Linda Abonyo
The National Council on Problem Gambling has affiliate organizations in most states. For a complete listing, go to http://www.ncpgambling.org/state_affiliates/

Compulsive Gambling Institute
27620 Landau Blvd., Suite 1B
Cathedral City, CA 92234
(760) 327-8880   Office
(760) 327-8804   FAX
(760) 902-3529   New Cell
www.gamblingaddiction.cc
Chief Executive Officer: Tom Tucker

Gamblers Anonymous
International Service Office
P.O. Box 17173, Los Angeles, CA 90017
(213) 386-8789 - Fax (213) 386-0030
Gamblers Anonymous has chapters throughout the world. The GA website, http://gamblersanonymous.org/, lists U.S. cities with chapters and how to contact them.

Bibliography

Asbury, Herbert. *Sucker's Progress: An Informal History of Gambling in America from the Colonies to Canfield.* Dodd, Mead and Company, 1938.

Barnes, Lee H. *Dummy Up and Deal: Inside the Culture of Casino Dealing.* University of Nevada Press, 2002

Barthelme, Frederick & Steve. *Double Down: The gripping account of a two-year gambling splurge and its aftermath.* Harcourt, Inc, 1999.

Bergler, Edmund, MD. *The Psychology of Gambling.* International Universities Press, Inc., 1958.

Bernstein, Peter L. *Against the Gods: The Remarkable Story of Risk.* John Wiley & Sons, 1996.

Brunner, Robert K. *Treasury of Gambling Stories,* Ziff Davis Publishing Company, 1946.

Castellani, Brian. *Pathological Gambling: The Making of a Medical Problem.* State University of New York Press, 2000.

Chafetz, Henry. *Play the Devil: A History of Gambling in the United States from 1492 to 1955.* Bonanza Books, 1960.

Cotton, Charles. *The Compleat Gamester.* (1674). Cornmarket, 1972.

Davis-Goff, Annabel. *The Literary Companion to Gambling.* Sinclair-Stevenson, 1996.

Denton, Sally & Morris, Roger. *The Money and the Power: The Making of Las Vegas and its Hold on America, 1947-2000.* Alfred A. Knopf, 2001

Dostoyevsky, Fyodor. *The Gambler.* (1866) Dover Publications, 1996.

Estes, Ken. *Deadly Odds: The Compulsion to Gamble.* Edgehill Publications, 1990.

Fabian, Ann. Card Sharps, *Dream Books & Bucket Shops: Gambling in 19th Century America.* Cornell University Press, 1990.

Findlay, John M. *People of Chance: Gambling in American Society from Jamestown to Las Vegas.* Oxford University Press, 1986.

Isaacs, Neil D. *You Bet Your Life: The Burdens of Gambling.* University of Kentucky Press, 2001.

Knapp, Bettina L. *Gambling, Game & Psyche*. State University of New York Press, 2000.

Lesieur, Henry R. *The Chase: The Compulsive Gambler*. Schenkman Books, Inc., 1984

Lorenz, Valerie C., Ph.D. *Releasing Guilt About Gambling*. Hazelden, 1993.

Lyons, Paul. *The Quotable Gambler*. The Lyons Press, 1999.

McGurrin, Martin C. *Pathological Gambling: Conceptual, Diagnostic, and Treatment Issues*. Professional Resource Press, 1992.

Nakken, Craig. The Addictive Personality: Understanding the Addictive Process and Compulsive Gambling. Hazelden, 1996.

O'Brien, Timothy. *Bad Bet: The Inside Story of the Glamour, Glitz, and Danger of America's Gambling Industy*. Random House, 1998.

Ore, Oystein. *Cardano: The Gambling Scholar*. Dover Publications, Inc., 1952.

Pietrusza, David. Rothstein: *The Life, Times, and Murder of the Criminal Genius Who Fixed the 1919 World Series*. Carroll & Graf Publishers, 2003.

Quinn, John Philip. *Fools of Fortune: or Gambling and Gamblers*. The Anti-Gambling Association, 1892.

Sharing Recovery Through Gamblers Anonymous, Gamblers Anonymous Publishing Inc., 1984

Smith, John L. *Running Scared: The Life and Treacherous Times of Las Vegas Casino King Steve Wynn*. Four Walls, Eight Windows, 2001.

Stuart, Lyle. *Casino Gambling for the Winner*. Ballentine Books, 1978.

Thackrey, Ted Jr. *Gambling Secrets of Nick the Greek*. Pocket Books, 1968.

Vogel, Jennifer. *Crapped Out: How Gambling Ruins the Economy and Destroys Lives*. Common Courage Press, 1997.

Wagner, Walter. *To Gamble or Not to Gamble: An Inquiry into the Personal and Social Costs of Money Games*. World Publishing, 1972

Weinberg, Robert. *The Revolution of 1905 in Odessa: Blood on the Steps*. Bloomington University Press, 1993.

About the Author

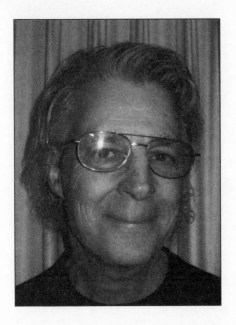

Burt Dragin teaches journalism at Laney College in Oakland, California. He has written for various newspapers and magazines. This is his first book. He lives in Berkeley with his wife Nadine, daughter Ana, one dog and two cats. He tries not to think about gambling. He can be contacted at burtdragin@aol.com.